Type 2 Diabetes Cookbook
Beginner's Quick & Easy Recipes for Delicious Diabetes Diets

300 Healthy

Sauces, Dips, and Dressings

for

Diabetic Wellness in 30 minutes or Less

By

Lily Anders

Copyright Page

Ace East Publishing LLC
1401 21st Street
Suite R
Sacramento, CA 95811

ISBN: **978-1-963939-83-5**

First Edition

ACE EAST PUBLISHING

Disclaimer Page

This cookbook is crafted to offer insightful information and recipes for those interested in managing Type 2 Diabetes through dietary choices. It is important to recognize that the authors and the publisher are not healthcare professionals. The suggestions and recipes contained within this book are not meant to replace professional medical advice, diagnoses, or treatments. Should you have any healthcare-related questions or concerns, particularly relating to Type 2 Diabetes management, we strongly advise consulting with your doctor or a qualified healthcare provider.

The culinary experiences, and recommendations shared in this book stem from extensive research and the personal journey of exploring dietary approaches to Type 2 Diabetes management. These narratives and suggestions are intended for educational and motivational purposes only, aiming to enhance understanding and inspire positive lifestyle changes, not to serve as direct medical or nutritional prescriptions.

The author(s) and publisher expressly disclaim any liability for any adverse effects arising directly or indirectly from the use and application of the information contained in this cookbook. Moreover, given the specificity and medical relevance of the content, certain topics and dietary advice may not be suitable for all readers. It is advisable for caregivers and adults to review the content before sharing with minors or individuals with particular sensitivities or health concerns.

In cases of medical emergencies or for immediate assistance with health issues, please reach out to a trusted healthcare professional or dial the emergency services number available in your locality.

The Entire Type 2 Diabetes Cookbook Series

Dive into a culinary revolution with the ***"Type 2 Diabetes Cookbook Series: Beginner's Quick & Easy Recipes for Delicious Diabetes Diets – 300 Health-Boosting Savory Meals for Diabetic Wellness in 30 Minutes or Less."***

Spread across six essential volumes – Breakfast, Lunch, Dinner, Desserts, Snacks, and Sauces, Dips, & Dressings – this series is your passport to a world where managing Type 2 Diabetes meets delicious innovation.

Each book is a treasure trove of hundreds of recipes, marrying the precision of nutritional science with the flair of culinary art. Designed for those on a diabetic diet, these recipes promise to transform your meals from bland to blissful without sacrificing flavor or health. Every dish, from energizing breakfasts to indulgent desserts, comes alive through vivid, full-color photographs, accompanied by foolproof instructions, cooking times, detailed ingredient lists, serving suggestions, and handy conversion charts.

But the journey doesn't end with tantalizing meals. These cookbooks are gateways to mastering diabetes management, offering insights into blood sugar balance, insulin functionality, and the art of carb counting. They stand as pillars of empowerment and knowledge, guiding you through the culinary and health aspects of diabetes with ease and enjoyment.

Embrace these cookbooks as more than mere collections of recipes; see them as companions in your journey toward diabetic wellness, bringing confidence, pleasure, and a burst of flavors into your daily life. Step into a world where managing diabetes is synonymous with culinary discovery and dietary joy. Welcome to your new kitchen adventure!

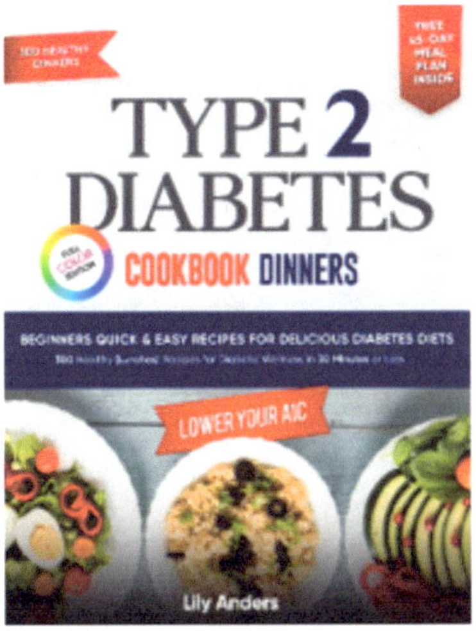
TYPE 2
DIABETES
COOKBOOK DINNERS
BEGINNERS QUICK & EASY RECIPES FOR DELICIOUS DIABETES DIETS
LOWER YOUR A1C
Lily Anders

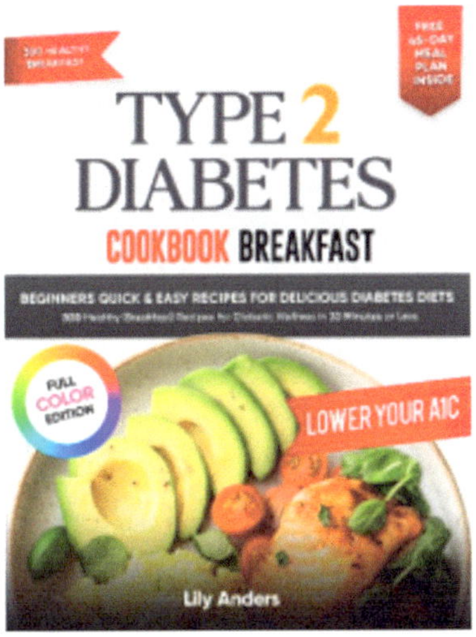
TYPE 2
DIABETES
COOKBOOK BREAKFAST
BEGINNERS QUICK & EASY RECIPES FOR DELICIOUS DIABETES DIETS
FULL COLOR EDITION
LOWER YOUR A1C
Lily Anders

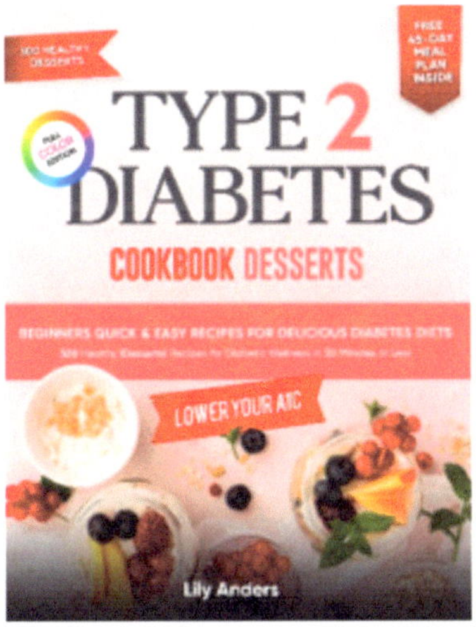
TYPE 2
DIABETES
COOKBOOK DESSERTS
LOWER YOUR A1C
Lily Anders

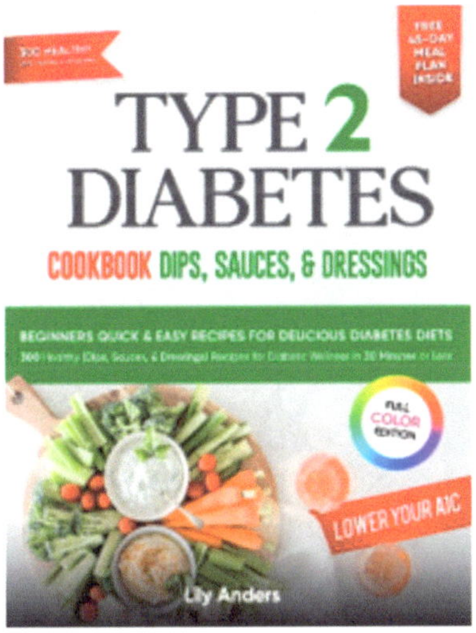
TYPE 2
DIABETES
COOKBOOK DIPS, SAUCES, & DRESSINGS
BEGINNERS QUICK & EASY RECIPES FOR DELICIOUS DIABETES DIETS
FULL COLOR EDITION
LOWER YOUR A1C
Lily Anders

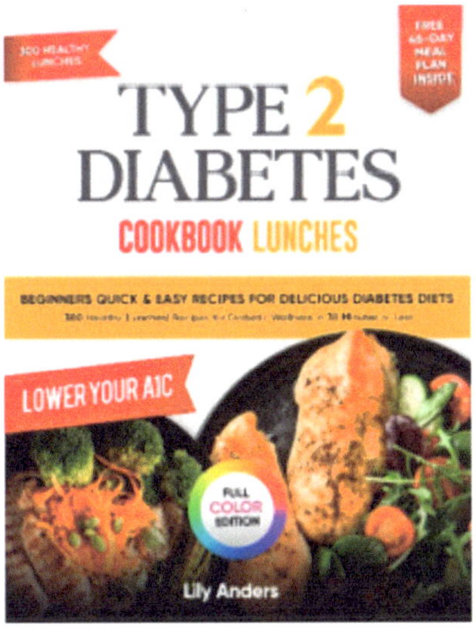
TYPE 2
DIABETES
COOKBOOK LUNCHES
BEGINNERS QUICK & EASY RECIPES FOR DELICIOUS DIABETES DIETS
LOWER YOUR A1C
FULL COLOR EDITION
Lily Anders

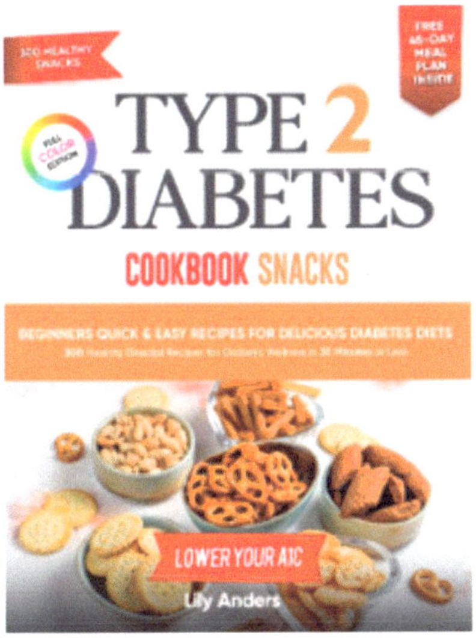
TYPE 2
DIABETES
COOKBOOK SNACKS
LOWER YOUR A1C
Lily Anders

Here's My Promise to You!

To jumpstart your journey toward healthier eating, here is the remaining

Listing of 200 Delicious & Diabetes-Friendly Sauces, Dips, & Dressings Recipes!

That's right—you now have access to a treasure trove of 200 additional diabetic recipes designed to help you enjoy flavorful, balanced meals while managing your blood sugar with confidence. These Sauces, Dips, & Dressings recipes will inspire you to create satisfying, nutritious meals with ease.

☞ CLICK here OR SCAN THE QR CODE TO DOWNLOAD YOUR FREE RECIPE COLLECTION!

Enjoy, and Happy Cooking!

The journey to better health starts with the right food choices, and this cookbook and it is here to support you every step of the way.

Thank you for trusting this guide, and here's to a flavorful, balanced, and empowered approach to managing Type 2 Diabetes!

You've got this! □□✨

<<Click here to access your 45-day meal plan>>
https://acrobat.adobe.com/id/urn:aaid:sc:VA6C2:448a7fa7-ffcd-4919-9d29-1c8e6bee62e9

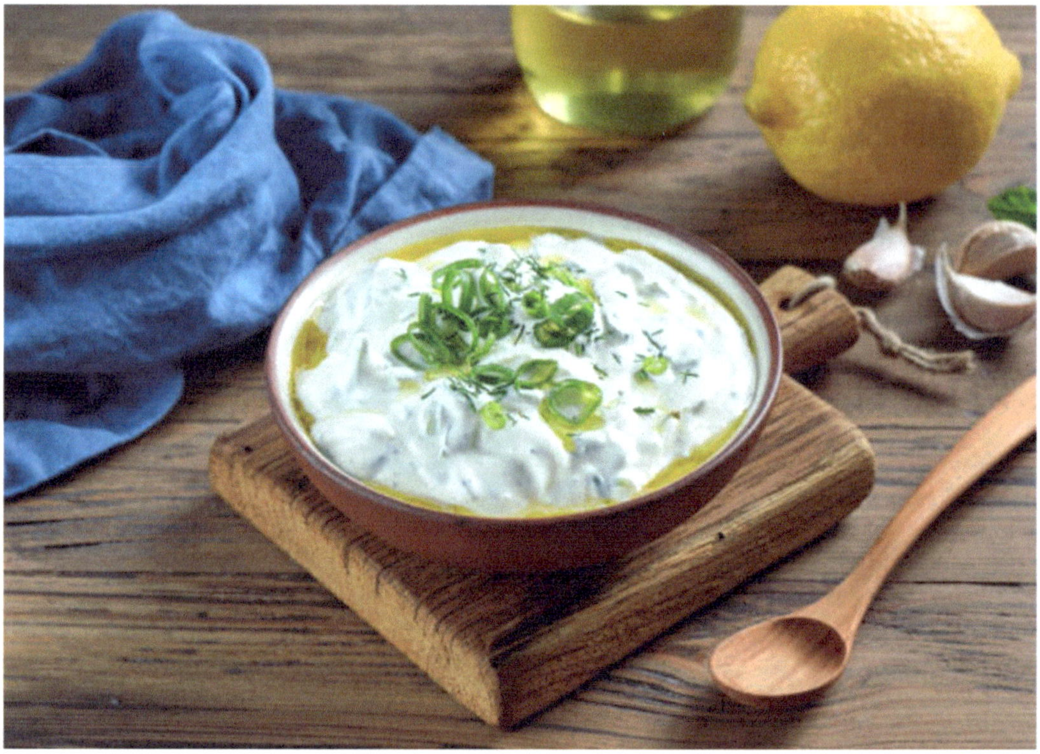

1. Greek Yogurt Tzatziki Sauce

Prep.Time: 10 min	**Cook Time:** 0 min	**Serving:** 4

Ingredients:

- 1 cup Greek yogurt (low-fat or non-fat)
- 1/2 cucumber, peeled, seeded, and finely chopped
- 1 clove garlic, minced
- 1 tablespoon lemon juice
- 1 tablespoon extra virgin olive oil
- 1 tablespoon chopped fresh dill (or 1 teaspoon dried dill)
- Salt and pepper to taste

Preparation:

1. In a mixing bowl, combine Greek yogurt, chopped cucumber, minced garlic, lemon juice, olive oil, and dill.
2. Stir well to combine.
3. Season with salt and pepper according to taste.
4. Refrigerate for at least 30 minutes before serving to allow flavors to meld.
5. Serve chilled with vegetables, pita bread, or as a topping for grilled meats.

Nutrient Facts (per serving):

- Calories: 60
- Carbohydrates: 4g
- Fat: 3g
- Protein: 5g

Table of Contents

INTRODUCTION

Where Flavor Meets Balance

For many people managing Type 2 Diabetes, meals begin with good intentions and end with hidden challenges. The protein is lean, the vegetables are fresh, and portions are reasonable. Yet blood sugar levels still feel unpredictable, and meals do not always deliver the results expected.

Often, the issue is not the meal itself.
It is what is added to it.

Sauces, dips, and dressings quietly shape the nutritional impact of food. They enhance flavor, bring meals together, and make eating enjoyable. They can also introduce unexpected sugars, refined carbohydrates, and excess calories that disrupt blood sugar balance without being obvious.

This book was written to address that hidden gap.

The Type 2 Diabetes Cookbook: Sauces, Dips, and Dressings focuses on flavor-forward additions designed to support blood sugar stability rather than undermine it. These recipes allow meals to feel complete and satisfying without relying on store-bought products that often contain unnecessary sugars and fillers.

Flavor is not the enemy. Lack of awareness is.

Sauces and dressings serve an important role in how food is experienced. When flavor is missing, meals feel restrictive and unsustainable. When flavor is added thoughtfully, healthy eating becomes easier to maintain.

Inside this book, you will find practical, diabetes-conscious recipes that complement breakfasts, lunches, dinners, and snacks throughout the day. Each option is designed to enhance meals without overwhelming them, using simple ingredients and balanced combinations.

This cookbook is not about eliminating condiments or eating plainly. It is about taking control of what is added to your food so that flavor works in your favor.

You will not need complicated techniques or specialty ingredients. These recipes are approachable, adaptable, and meant for everyday use.

When sauces and dressings support your goals, meals become more enjoyable and more consistent.

Welcome to a smarter, more confident way to add flavor to your life.

Chapter 1

Understanding Type 2 Diabetes and Hidden Sugars

Hidden sugars are one of the most common and frustrating challenges for individuals managing Type 2 Diabetes. Meals may appear balanced on the plate, yet blood sugar levels behave unpredictably. Often, the cause is not the main ingredients, but the sauces, dips, and dressings added for flavor.

Type 2 Diabetes affects how the body processes glucose. Insulin helps move glucose from the bloodstream into the cells, but when insulin function is impaired, glucose remains in the blood longer than intended. Foods that digest quickly or contain added sugars can intensify this effect.

Hidden sugars make this process harder to recognize and manage.

Where Hidden Sugars Commonly Appear

Many store-bought sauces and dressings contain added sugars, even when they do not taste sweet. Ingredients such as syrups, concentrates, and sweeteners are often used to enhance flavor, improve texture, or extend shelf life.

Salad dressings, marinades, dipping sauces, and condiments are frequent sources of these hidden sugars. Because they are used in small amounts, they are often overlooked. However, when combined with meals, they can significantly increase total carbohydrate intake.

These additions can quietly shift a balanced meal into one that disrupts blood sugar stability.

Why Hidden Sugars Matter More Than Expected

Sauces and dressings are typically consumed alongside other carbohydrates. When hidden sugars are added on top of grains, fruits, or starchy vegetables, the combined effect can lead to sharper blood sugar rises.

Because these sugars digest quickly, they may cause spikes that feel unexpected or confusing. This can lead to frustration, especially when efforts have been made to choose balanced meals.

Understanding where sugars hide allows you to regain control.

Reading Ingredient Lists with Awareness

Ingredient lists provide valuable information, but they can be misleading without context. Sugar may appear under many names, including syrups, concentrates, and sweeteners that sound natural or healthy.

The order of ingredients also matters. Ingredients listed earlier appear in greater amounts. When sugars or sweeteners are listed near the top, it is a sign that the product may significantly impact blood sugar levels.

Learning to scan labels with intention helps identify products that may not support your goals.

The Impact of Frequency and Portion Size

Even small amounts of sugar can add up when used frequently. Sauces and dressings are often added generously and repeatedly throughout the day.

Portion size matters, but frequency matters as well. Using multiple sugar-containing condiments in one meal can amplify their effect.

Being mindful of both how much and how often sauces are used supports better blood sugar management.

Moving From Awareness to Action

The purpose of this chapter is not to create fear around flavor. It is to build awareness so that sauces and dressings can be chosen intentionally.

As you begin to recognize where hidden sugars appear, it becomes easier to make adjustments. These adjustments do not require giving up flavor. They require understanding how to add flavor in ways that support balance.

In the next chapter, we will explore how blood sugar responds to sauces and dressings, and why small changes in ingredients and portions can make a meaningful difference.

Chapter 2

Blood Sugar Impact of Sauces and Condiments

Sauces and condiments often seem insignificant because they are used in small amounts. Yet their impact on blood sugar can be meaningful, especially when they are used frequently or combined with other carbohydrate-containing foods. Understanding this impact helps explain why some meals affect blood sugar more than expected.

For individuals managing Type 2 Diabetes, awareness of how sauces interact with meals is an important part of building consistency.

How Sauces Influence Blood Sugar Response

Sauces and condiments often contain added sugars or refined carbohydrates that digest quickly. When these are added to a meal, they increase the total carbohydrate load, sometimes without being obvious.

Because sauces are typically consumed alongside other foods, their sugars are absorbed at the same time as carbohydrates from grains, fruits, or vegetables. This combined intake can lead to higher or faster blood sugar rises than anticipated.

Even when the main components of a meal are balanced, sauces can change how the body responds.

The Cumulative Effect of Small Additions

A single tablespoon of sauce may not seem impactful, but multiple additions can add up quickly. A meal may include dressing on a salad, sauce on a protein, and a dip on the side.

Each addition contributes to the overall carbohydrate and sugar intake. Over time, these cumulative effects can make blood sugar patterns feel unpredictable.

Recognizing the combined impact of sauces helps explain why meals sometimes feel more challenging to manage.

Timing and Blood Sugar Stability

The timing of sauce consumption matters. Sauces consumed with meals may have a different effect than those eaten alone or added to snacks.

When sauces are paired with protein, fiber, and healthy fats, their impact on blood sugar may be moderated. When sauces are used heavily on refined carbohydrates, their sugars may digest more quickly.

Understanding this interaction allows for more thoughtful pairing and portion control.

Emotional and Habitual Use of Sauces

Sauces often serve as comfort or habit rather than necessity. They add familiarity and enjoyment, which is important, but habitual use can lead to larger portions than intended.

Pouring rather than measuring, dipping repeatedly, or adding sauces automatically can increase intake without awareness. These habits are common and understandable.

Becoming mindful of how sauces are used helps support balance without eliminating enjoyment.

Making Sauces Work for You

The goal is not to remove sauces from meals. It is to choose and use them in ways that support blood sugar stability.

Selecting sauces with lower sugar content, using smaller portions, and pairing them thoughtfully allows flavor to enhance meals without undermining balance.

This approach turns sauces from a hidden challenge into a supportive element of eating well.

In the next chapter, we will explore carbohydrates in sauces and dressings, focusing on how to choose ingredients and combinations that provide flavor without unnecessary excess.

Chapter 3

Carbohydrates in Sauces Without Overload

Carbohydrates in sauces, dips, and dressings are often underestimated. Because these items are used to enhance meals rather than serve as the main component, their carbohydrate content can feel insignificant. In reality, these carbohydrates can meaningfully affect blood sugar when used frequently or in generous amounts.

Understanding how carbohydrates appear in sauces allows flavor to remain enjoyable without overwhelming balance.

Where Carbohydrates Enter Sauces

Carbohydrates in sauces typically come from sugars, starches, and thickening agents. Sweeteners are commonly added to balance acidity or enhance flavor. Starches may be used to improve texture or consistency.

Even ingredients that sound wholesome can contribute carbohydrates. Fruit concentrates, honey, and syrups all add sweetness but are digested quickly. Flour or cornstarch used as thickeners can also raise carbohydrate content.

Recognizing these sources helps explain why sauces can impact blood sugar more than expected.

Quality and Quantity Matter Together

Not all carbohydrates behave the same way. Small amounts of carbohydrates paired with fats, acids, and proteins often digest more slowly than refined sugars alone.

The issue arises when sauces rely heavily on refined carbohydrates and are used liberally. In these cases, both the quality and quantity of carbohydrates can create overload.

Choosing sauces that emphasize fats, herbs, spices, and acidity rather than sweetness helps reduce carbohydrate impact while maintaining flavor.

Portion Awareness With Sauces

Because sauces are often poured or dipped without measurement, portions can increase quickly. What begins as a small addition can become several servings over the course of a meal.

Using portion awareness with sauces is especially important. Serving sauces on the side or using a spoon rather than pouring directly helps maintain control.

Smaller portions can still deliver flavor when sauces are well-balanced and concentrated.

Pairing Sauces With Meals

How sauces are paired with meals influences their effect. Sauces added to protein-rich foods or vegetables tend to have a gentler impact on blood sugar than those used heavily on refined carbohydrates.

For example, a sauce paired with grilled vegetables or lean protein may support balance, while the same sauce poured over refined grains may contribute to overload.

Pairing choices matter as much as ingredient choices.

Redefining Sauce Expectations

Sauces do not need to be sweet to be satisfying. Savory, tangy, and herb-forward flavors can provide depth without relying on carbohydrates.

Redefining what a sauce should taste like allows for creativity and balance. When sweetness is used intentionally and sparingly, it enhances rather than dominates.

The recipes in this book are designed to demonstrate how carbohydrates can be included thoughtfully, allowing sauces to support meals instead of overwhelming them.

In the next chapter, we will focus on smart shopping strategies for sauces, dips, and dressings, helping you choose ingredients that make balanced flavor easier to achieve.

Chapter 4

Smart Sauce Shopping

Shopping for sauces, dips, and dressings can feel deceptively simple. Shelves are filled with options labeled as natural, light, or sugar-free, yet many of these products still contain ingredients that can disrupt blood sugar balance. Smart sauce shopping helps remove confusion and puts control back in your hands.

This chapter focuses on choosing flavor additions that support consistency rather than undermine it.

Reading Labels With Purpose

Ingredient lists are the most reliable source of information when shopping for sauces. Marketing claims on the front of packaging can be misleading, while the ingredient list reveals what is truly inside.

Look for short, recognizable ingredient lists. Sauces built around oils, vinegar, herbs, spices, and whole ingredients tend to be more supportive than those relying on added sugars or refined starches.

Be mindful of the many names used for sugar, including syrups, concentrates, and sweeteners that sound natural. When these appear early in the ingredient list, the product is likely higher in carbohydrates than expected.

Understanding Serving Sizes

Sauce labels often list small serving sizes that do not reflect how products are commonly used. A single serving may appear reasonable, yet typical portions can be several times larger.

When reviewing nutrition information, consider how much you are likely to use rather than relying solely on the listed serving size. This perspective provides a more accurate understanding of how a product may affect blood sugar.

Awareness of serving size helps prevent unintentional excess.

Choosing Sauces That Support Balance

Sauces that emphasize fats, acids, and savory flavors often have a gentler impact on blood sugar. Oil-based dressings, vinegar-forward sauces, and herb-rich dips provide depth without relying heavily on carbohydrates.

Products that list sugar or refined starches as primary ingredients are more likely to contribute to blood sugar fluctuations. Choosing alternatives with minimal added sugars helps maintain balance.

When possible, selecting unsweetened or lightly sweetened options provides greater flexibility and control.

Shopping for Versatility

Versatile ingredients simplify shopping and reduce reliance on multiple products. Oils, vinegars, mustards, herbs, spices, and plain yogurt can be used to create a wide range of sauces and dressings at home.

Having these staples on hand allows you to adjust flavors without introducing unnecessary sugars. This approach also reduces dependency on store-bought products with long ingredient lists.

Versatility supports both creativity and consistency.

Making Sauce Shopping Sustainable

Effective sauce shopping becomes easier with familiarity. As you identify dependable products and ingredients, shopping becomes faster and more intuitive.

Over time, your pantry begins to reflect your goals, making balanced meals easier to prepare without constant label scrutiny.

In the next chapter, we will explore preparation strategies that make sauces, dips, and dressings easy to create and use, helping flavor fit naturally into your daily routine.

Chapter 5

Prep Strategies for Flavor Without Sugar

Creating flavorful sauces, dips, and dressings does not require added sugar. In many cases, sugar is used as a shortcut rather than a necessity. With a few intentional preparation strategies, flavor can be built through balance, texture, and contrast instead.

These strategies help make sauces supportive of blood sugar stability while still enhancing meals.

Building Flavor With Core Elements

Flavor comes from a combination of fat, acid, salt, and aroma. Oils provide richness and mouthfeel, acids such as vinegar or citrus add brightness, and salt enhances natural flavors. Herbs, spices, garlic, and onions add depth and complexity.

When these elements are balanced, sweetness is often unnecessary. For example, acidity can brighten a sauce, while fats help carry flavor and create satisfaction.

Learning to rely on these core elements allows sauces to feel complete without sugar.

Preparing Base Sauces in Advance

Preparing simple base sauces ahead of time reduces reliance on store-bought options. A basic vinaigrette, yogurt-based dressing, or oil-and-herb blend can be stored and used across multiple meals.

These base sauces can be adjusted easily with different herbs, spices, or acids, creating variety without extra effort. Preparing bases once and using them throughout the week saves time and supports consistency.

Advance preparation makes flavorful choices easier on busy days.

Using Natural Flavor Enhancers

Natural flavor enhancers such as roasted garlic, caramelized onions, herbs, spices, and citrus zest add richness without sugar. These ingredients deepen flavor and provide complexity.

Cooking techniques such as roasting, grilling, or sautéing can also enhance natural sweetness in vegetables without adding sugar. These methods allow flavors to develop through heat rather than through sweeteners.

Using these techniques helps sauces feel satisfying and well-rounded.

Keeping Portions Balanced During Preparation

Because sugar-free sauces rely on concentrated flavors, smaller portions are often sufficient. Preparing sauces with balance in mind helps prevent overuse.

Serving sauces on the side allows control over portion size and encourages mindful use. This approach helps flavor enhance the meal without dominating it.

Portion awareness during preparation supports both taste and balance.

Creating a Sustainable Flavor Routine

The most effective preparation strategies are repeatable and realistic. Keeping a short list of dependable sauces and dips makes it easier to add flavor consistently.

Over time, these sauces become part of your routine, reducing the need for processed condiments and supporting blood sugar-friendly meals.

Flavor should make healthy eating easier, not more complicated.

In the next chapter, we will focus on portion awareness for sauces, dips, and dressings, helping you enjoy flavor without unintentionally increasing carbohydrate intake.

Chapter 6

Portion Awareness for Sauces and Dressings

Portion size plays a quiet but powerful role in how sauces, dips, and dressings affect blood sugar. Even thoughtfully prepared, low-sugar options can disrupt balance when used in excess. Portion awareness allows flavor to enhance meals without unintentionally increasing carbohydrate intake.

This chapter focuses on using sauces intentionally, so they support consistency rather than create confusion.

Why Sauce Portions Matter

Sauces and dressings are often concentrated sources of flavor. Because they are added rather than eaten on their own, it is easy to use more than intended. Small increases in portion size can significantly change the nutritional impact of a meal.

For individuals managing Type 2 Diabetes, frequent or generous use of sauces can add carbohydrates and calories that go unnoticed. Over time, this can affect blood sugar patterns and make meals feel less predictable.

Portion awareness helps restore clarity.

Recognizing Appropriate Sauce Portions

A supportive portion of sauce is usually smaller than expected. One or two tablespoons are often enough to add flavor without overwhelming the meal.

Serving sauces on the side rather than pouring them directly onto food allows you to control how much is used. Dipping lightly rather than coating food helps maintain balance while still delivering flavor.

Visual cues can be helpful. A small spoon or ramekin provides a clear boundary that supports portion awareness.

Common Portion Pitfalls

One of the most common challenges with sauces is automatic use. Pouring without measuring, dipping repeatedly, or adding sauce to every component of a meal can quickly increase intake.

Another common pattern is compensating for bland food by adding more sauce. Improving the base flavors of meals often reduces the need for larger sauce portions.

Awareness of these habits allows for simple adjustments without eliminating enjoyment.

Pairing Sauces With Intention

How sauces are paired with meals influences their effect. Sauces used with vegetables or protein generally have a gentler impact than those added heavily to refined carbohydrates.

Using sauce strategically, rather than evenly across the plate, helps flavor stand out while keeping portions controlled. This approach allows meals to remain satisfying without excess.

Building Long-Term Confidence With Flavor

As portion awareness improves, using sauces becomes more intuitive. You begin to recognize how much is enough and how different sauces affect your body.

The recipes in this book are designed with portion awareness in mind, helping remove guesswork while preserving enjoyment.

When sauces, dips, and dressings are used intentionally, they become powerful tools that make balanced eating more enjoyable and sustainable.

In the next section, we will transition into the recipes, where these principles are applied through practical, flavorful additions designed to complement meals throughout the day.

Letting Flavor Work for You

The guidance you have explored in this section is meant to shift how you think about flavor, not to limit it. Understanding hidden sugars, learning how sauces influence blood sugar, and developing practical habits around shopping, preparation, and portion awareness all serve one purpose, to help flavor support your goals rather than quietly undermine them.

Now it is time to put those principles into practice.

The recipes that follow are designed to enhance meals without adding unnecessary sugars or carbohydrates. Each sauce, dip, and dressing emphasizes balance, simplicity, and intention, allowing flavor to elevate your food while respecting blood sugar stability. These recipes are meant to complement breakfasts, lunches, dinners, and snacks throughout the day.

You do not need to prepare every recipe or use them all at once. Choose options that fit your preferences and your routine. Some will become everyday staples, while others may be reserved for specific meals or occasions. Both uses are encouraged.

As you explore the recipes, pay attention to how small additions affect both flavor and balance. Use that awareness to guide portion size and pairing choices that feel sustainable and satisfying.

This section is not about eating plainly or giving up enjoyment. It is about reclaiming control over what is added to your meals, so flavor becomes an ally rather than a hidden obstacle.

Let these recipes help you finish meals feeling confident, satisfied, and supported.

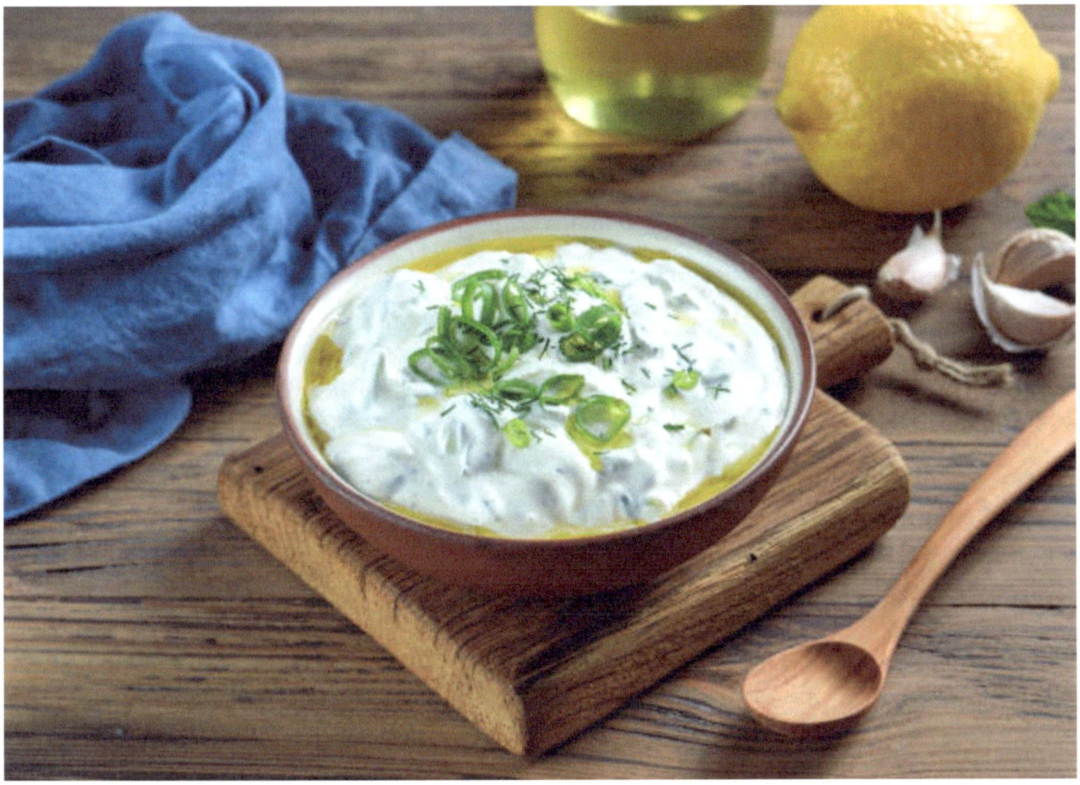

1. Greek Yogurt Tzatziki Sauce

Prep.Time: 10 min | **Cook Time:** 0 min | **Serving:** 4

Ingredients:

- 1 cup Greek yogurt (low-fat or non-fat)
- 1/2 cucumber, peeled, seeded, and finely chopped
- 1 clove garlic, minced
- 1 tablespoon lemon juice
- 1 tablespoon extra virgin olive oil
- 1 tablespoon chopped fresh dill (or 1 teaspoon dried dill)
- Salt and pepper to taste

Preparation:

1. In a mixing bowl, combine Greek yogurt, chopped cucumber, minced garlic, lemon juice, olive oil, and dill.
2. Stir well to combine.
3. Season with salt and pepper according to taste.
4. Refrigerate for at least 30 minutes before serving to allow flavors to meld.
5. Serve chilled with vegetables, pita bread, or as a topping for grilled meats.

Nutrient Facts (per serving):

- Calories: 60
- Carbohydrates: 4g
- Fat: 3g
- Protein: 5g

2. Butternut Squash Sage Sauce

Prep.Time: 40 min

Cook Time: 10 min

Serving: 4

Ingredients:

- 2 cups butternut squash, peeled and diced
- 2 tablespoons olive oil
- 2 cloves garlic, minced
- 1 tablespoon fresh sage leaves, chopped
- 1 cup vegetable broth
- Salt and pepper to taste
- Grated Parmesan cheese for garnish (optional)

Preparation:

1. Heat olive oil in a large skillet over medium heat. Add minced garlic and chopped sage leaves. Cook until fragrant, about 1 minute.
2. Add diced butternut squash to the skillet and sauté for 5-7 minutes until slightly softened.
3. Pour in the vegetable broth and bring to a simmer. Reduce the heat to low, cover, and let it cook for about 20-25 minutes, or until the butternut squash is tender.
4. Use a blender or immersion blender to puree the mixture until smooth. If the sauce is too thick, you can add more vegetable broth to reach the desired consistency.
5. Season with salt and pepper to taste.
6. Serve the butternut squash sage sauce over cooked pasta, gnocchi, or roasted vegetables.
7. Garnish with grated Parmesan cheese if desired.

Nutrient Facts (per serving):

- Calories: 120
- Carbohydrates: 20g
- Fat: 5g
- Protein: 2g

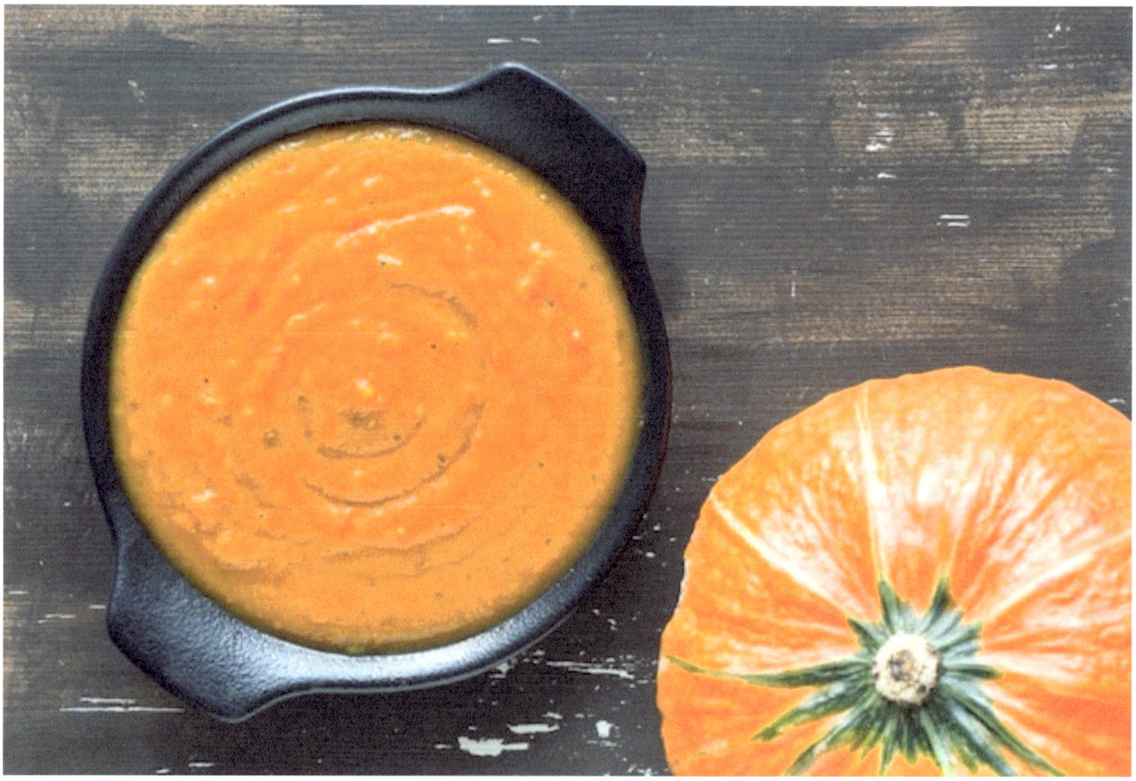

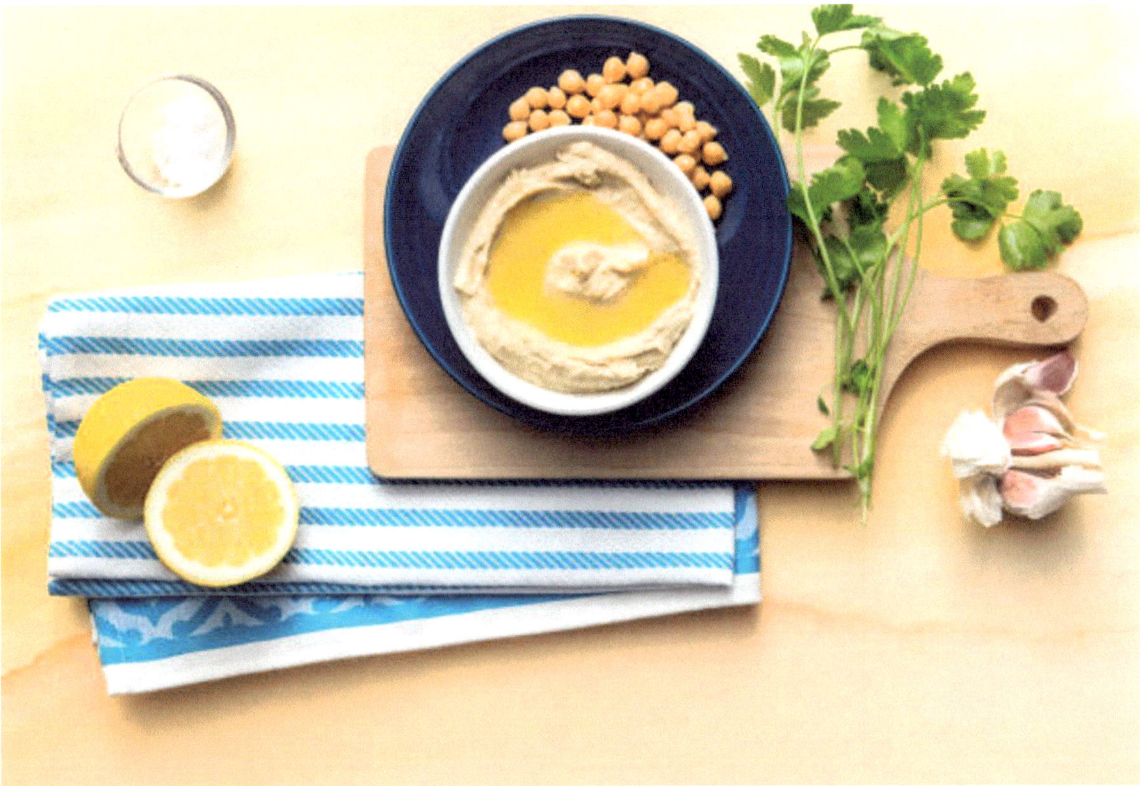

3. Hummus with Lemon and Garlic

Prep.Time: 10 min | **Cook Time:** 0 min | **Serving:** 4

Ingredients:

- 1 can (15 ounces) chickpeas (garbanzo beans), drained and rinsed
- 2 tablespoons tahini (sesame seed paste)
- 1 clove garlic, minced
- 2 tablespoons lemon juice
- 2 tablespoons extra virgin olive oil
- 1/2 teaspoon ground cumin
- Salt and pepper to taste
- Water (as needed for desired consistency)

Preparation:

1. In a food processor, combine chickpeas, tahini, minced garlic, lemon juice, olive oil, ground cumin, salt, and pepper.
2. Blend until smooth, scraping down the sides of the processor as needed.
3. If the hummus is too thick, add water, 1 tablespoon at a time, until desired consistency is reached.
4. Taste and adjust seasoning if necessary.
5. Transfer the hummus to a serving bowl.
6. Drizzle with a little extra olive oil and sprinkle with a pinch of cumin, if desired.
7. Serve with vegetable sticks, whole grain pita bread, or as a spread for sandwiches.

Nutrient Facts (per serving):

- Calories: 70
- Carbohydrates: 8g
- Fat: 3g
- Protein: 3g

4. Balsamic Vinaigrette Dressing

Prep.Time:	Cook Time:	Serving:
5 min	0 min	4

Ingredients:

- 3 tablespoons balsamic vinegar
- 2 tablespoons extra virgin olive oil
- 1 teaspoon Dijon mustard
- 1 clove garlic, minced
- Salt and pepper to taste

Preparation:

1. In a small bowl, whisk together balsamic vinegar, olive oil, Dijon mustard, and minced garlic until well combined.
2. Season with salt and pepper according to taste.
3. Taste and adjust seasoning if necessary.
4. Serve immediately over salads or as a marinade for grilled vegetables or meats.

Nutrient Facts (per serving):

- Calories: 50
- Carbohydrates: 4g
- Fat: 4g
- Protein: 0g

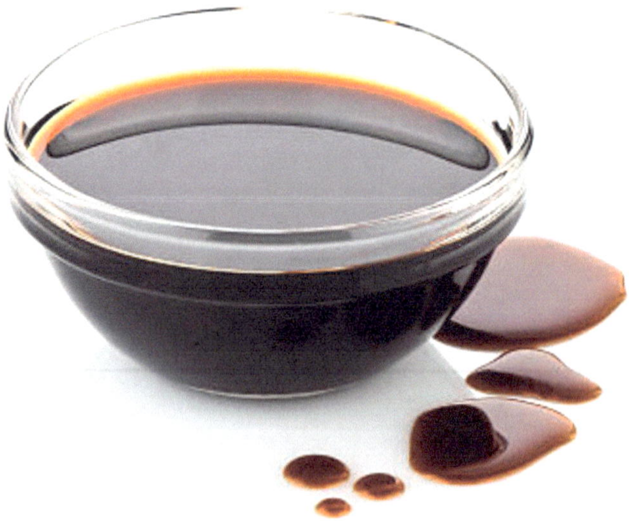

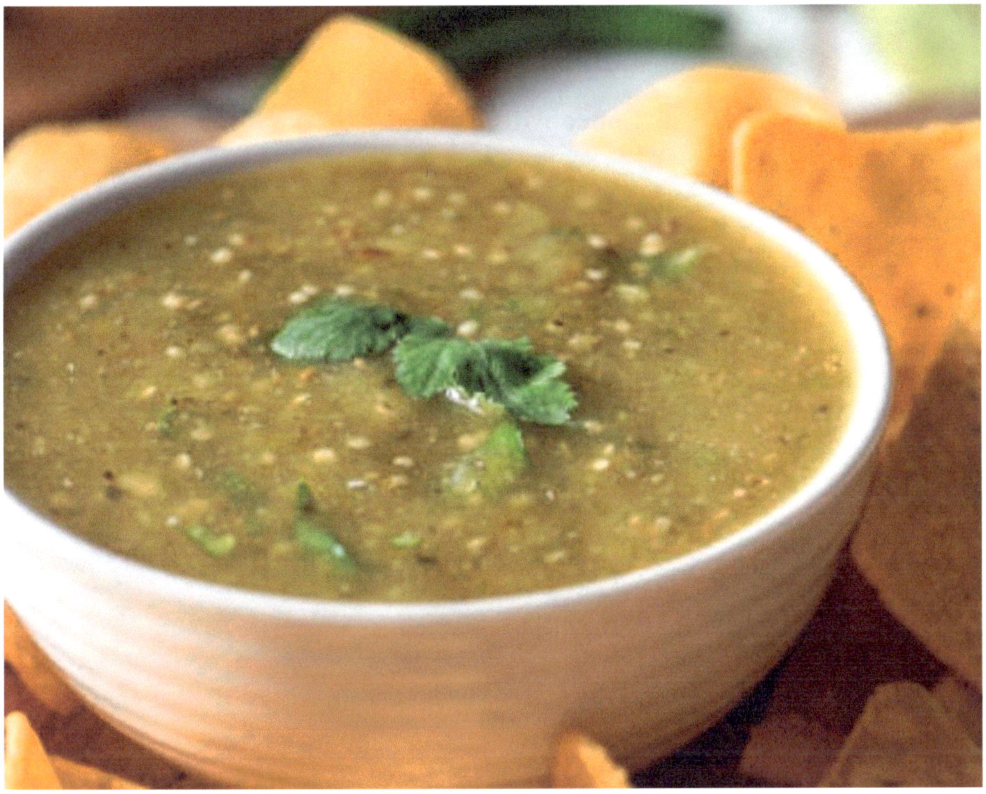

5. Salsa Verde with Roasted Tomatillos

Prep.Time: 15 min

Cook Time: 15 min

Serving: 4

Ingredients:

- 6 tomatillos, husks removed and rinsed
- 1 jalapeño pepper, stemmed and seeded
- 1/4 cup chopped onion
- 1/4 cup chopped fresh cilantro
- 1 clove garlic, minced
- 1 tablespoon lime juice
- Salt to taste

Preparation:

1. Preheat the broiler in your oven.
2. Place the tomatillos and jalapeño pepper on a baking sheet.
3. Broil for about 5-7 minutes, turning halfway through, until charred and softened.
4. Remove from the oven and let cool slightly.
5. In a blender or food processor, combine roasted tomatillos, jalapeño pepper, chopped onion, minced garlic, chopped cilantro, and lime juice.
6. Blend until smooth.
7. Season with salt to taste.
8. Transfer to a serving bowl.
9. Serve with tortilla chips, grilled chicken, fish, or use as a sauce for tacos or enchiladas.

Nutrient Facts (per serving):

- Calories: 30
- Carbohydrates: 4g
- Fat: 1g
- Protein: 1g

6. Pesto Sauce with Basil and Pine Nuts

Prep.Time: 10 min | **Cook Time:** 0 min | **Serving:** 4

Ingredients:

- 2 cups fresh basil leaves, packed
- 1/4 cup pine nuts
- 1/4 cup grated Parmesan cheese
- 1 clove garlic, minced
- 1/4 cup extra virgin olive oil
- Salt and pepper to taste

Preparation:

1. In a food processor, combine basil leaves, pine nuts, grated Parmesan cheese, and minced garlic.
2. Pulse until finely chopped.
3. While the food processor is running, gradually add the olive oil in a steady stream until the mixture is smooth and well combined.
4. Season with salt and pepper according to taste.
5. Taste and adjust seasoning if necessary.
6. Transfer the pesto sauce to a serving bowl.
7. Serve with whole grain pasta, zucchini noodles, grilled vegetables, or as a spread for sandwiches.

Nutrient Facts (per serving):

- Calories: 120
- Carbohydrates: 2g
- Fat: 12g
- Protein: 2g

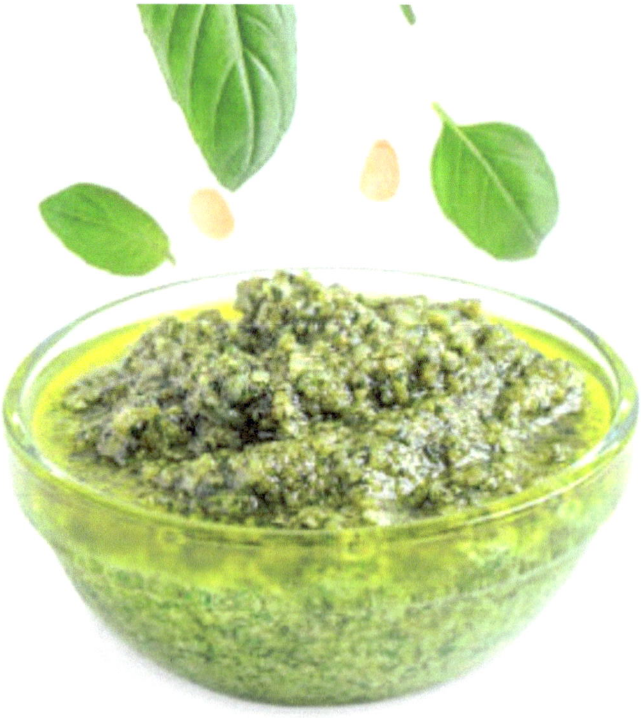

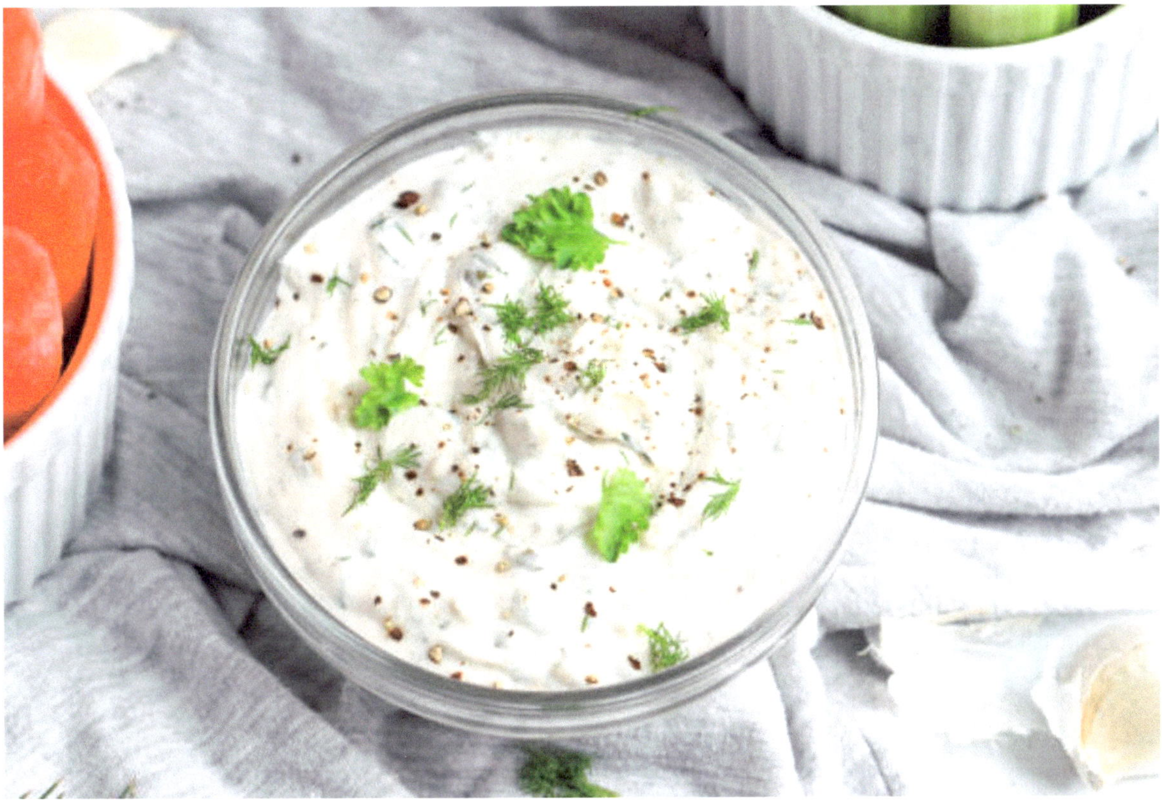

7. Ranch Dip with Greek Yogurt

Prep.Time: 10 min

Cook Time: 0 min

Serving: 4

Ingredients:

- 1 cup Greek yogurt (low-fat or non-fat)
- 1 tablespoon chopped fresh dill
- 1 tablespoon chopped fresh parsley
- 1 clove garlic, minced
- 1 teaspoon onion powder
- 1 teaspoon dried chives
- 1 teaspoon lemon juice
- Salt and pepper to taste

Preparation:

1. In a mixing bowl, combine Greek yogurt, chopped dill, chopped parsley, minced garlic, onion powder, dried chives, and lemon juice.
2. Stir well to combine.
3. Season with salt and pepper according to taste.
4. Refrigerate for at least 30 minutes before serving to allow flavors to meld.
5. Serve chilled with vegetable sticks, whole grain crackers, or as a dip for grilled meats.

Nutrient Facts (per serving):

- Calories: 40
- Carbohydrates: 2g
- Fat: 3g
- Protein: 2g

8. Sugar-Free BBQ Sauce

Prep.Time: 10 min | **Cook Time:** 15 min | **Serving:** 4

Ingredients:

- 1 cup tomato sauce (no sugar added)
- 2 tablespoons apple cider vinegar
- 1 tablespoon Worcestershire sauce (check for sugar-free version)
- 1 tablespoon Dijon mustard
- 1 teaspoon smoked paprika
- 1/2 teaspoon garlic powder
- 1/2 teaspoon onion powder
- Salt and pepper to taste
- Liquid stevia (optional, to taste)

Preparation:

1. In a saucepan, combine tomato sauce, apple cider vinegar, Worcestershire sauce, Dijon mustard, smoked paprika, garlic powder, and onion powder.
2. Stir well to combine.
3. Bring the mixture to a simmer over medium heat.
4. Reduce the heat to low and let the sauce simmer for about 10-15 minutes, stirring occasionally, until it thickens slightly.
5. Season with salt and pepper according to taste.
6. If desired, add liquid stevia to sweeten the sauce to your liking.
7. Remove from heat and let cool before serving.
8. Use as a marinade or glaze for grilled meats, or as a dipping sauce for vegetables.

Nutrient Facts (per serving):

- Calories: 20
- Carbohydrates: 4g
- Fat: 0g
- Protein: 1g

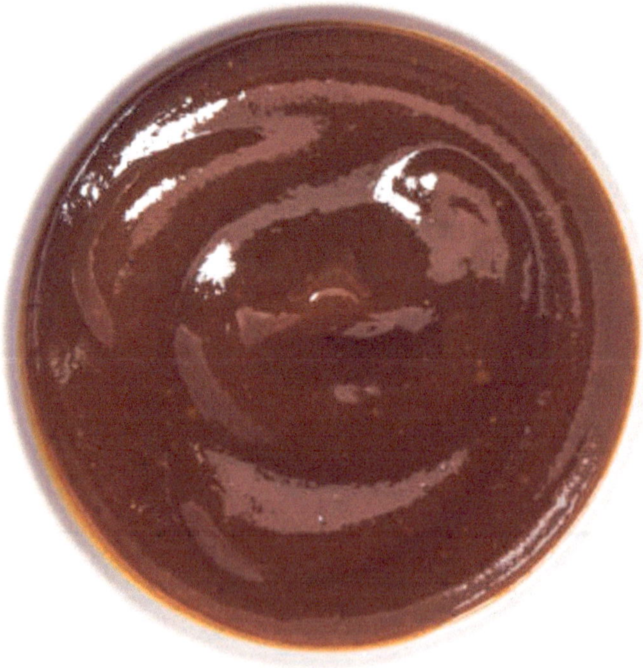

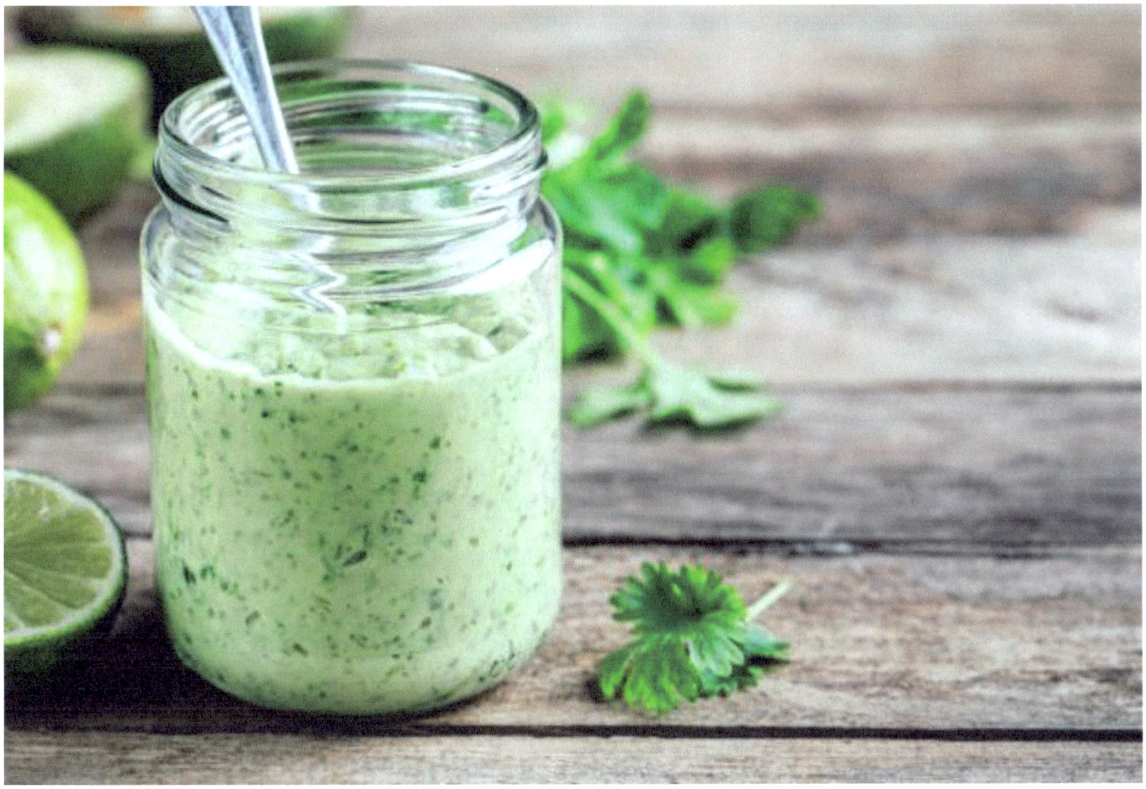

9. Cilantro Lime Dressing

Prep.Time: 5 min | **Cook Time:** 0 min | **Serving:** 4

Ingredients:

- 1/4 cup extra virgin olive oil
- 2 tablespoons lime juice
- 2 tablespoons chopped fresh cilantro
- 1 clove garlic, minced
- 1/2 teaspoon ground cumin
- Salt and pepper to taste

Preparation:

1. In a small bowl, whisk together extra virgin olive oil, lime juice, chopped cilantro, minced garlic, and ground cumin until well combined.
2. Season with salt and pepper according to taste.
3. Taste and adjust seasoning if necessary.
4. Serve immediately over salads or grilled vegetables.

Nutrient Facts (per serving):

- Calories: 60
- Carbohydrates: 2g
- Fat: 6g
- Protein: 1g

10. Cucumber and Dill Yogurt Dip

Prep.Time: 10 min | **Cook Time:** 0 min | **Serving:** 4

Ingredients:

- 1 cup Greek yogurt (low-fat or non-fat)
- 1/2 cucumber, peeled, seeded, and finely chopped
- 1 tablespoon chopped fresh dill
- 1 clove garlic, minced
- 1 teaspoon lemon juice
- Salt and pepper to taste

Preparation:

1. In a mixing bowl, combine Greek yogurt, chopped cucumber, chopped dill, minced garlic, and lemon juice.
2. Stir well to combine.
3. Season with salt and pepper according to taste.
4. Refrigerate for at least 30 minutes before serving to allow flavors to meld.
5. Serve chilled with vegetable sticks, whole grain crackers, or as a topping for grilled meats or fish.

Nutrient Facts (per serving):

- Calories: 30
- Carbohydrates: 3g
- Fat: 1g
- Protein: 2g

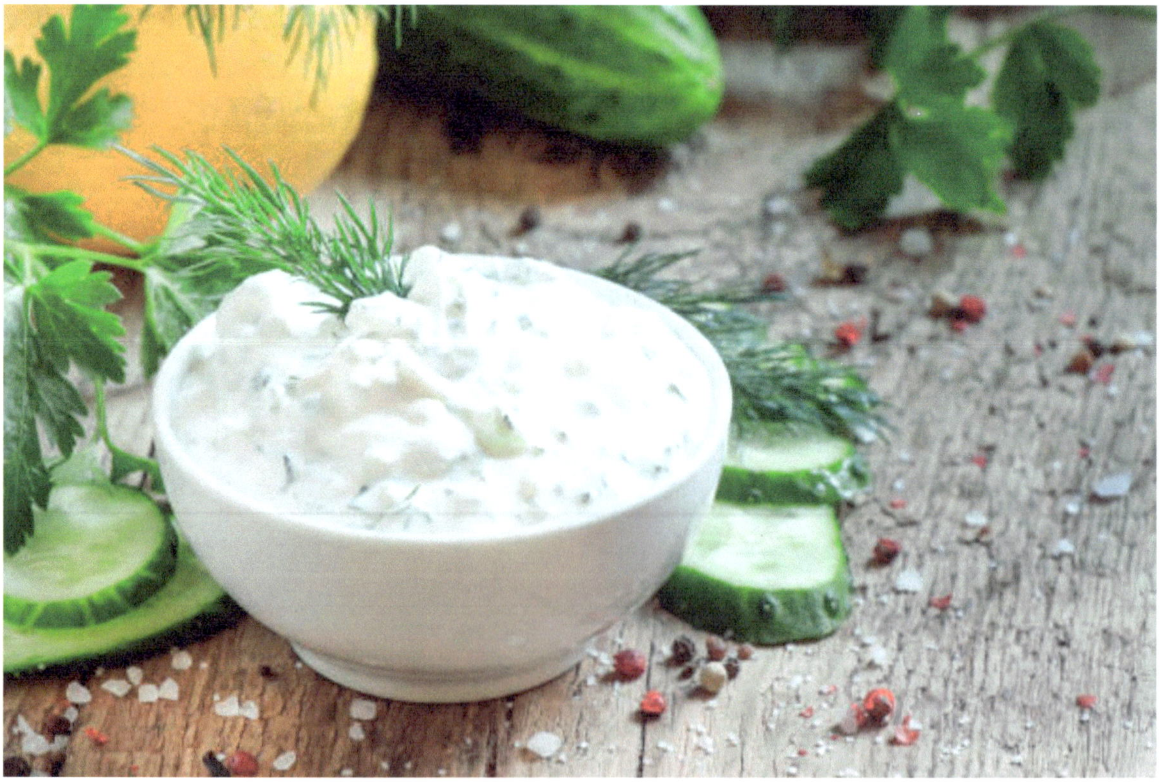

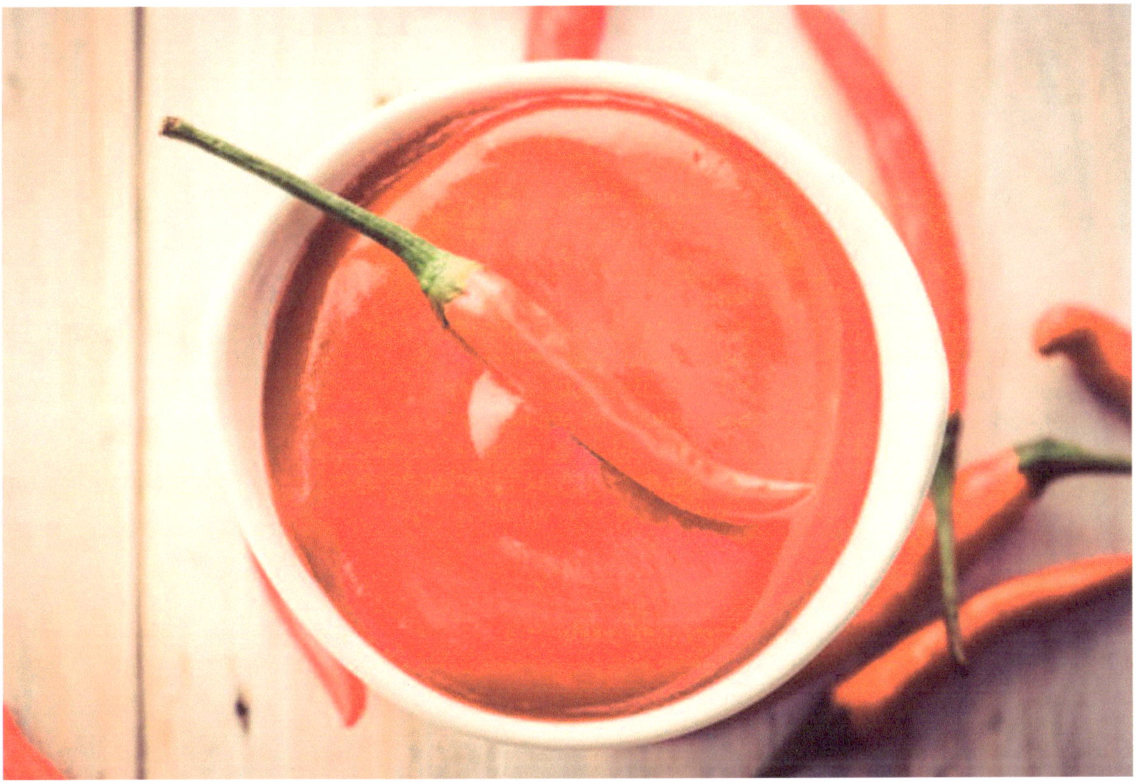

11. Spicy Sriracha Mayo

Prep.Time: 5 min

Cook Time: 0 min

Serving: 4

Ingredients:

- 1/2 cup mayonnaise (light or low-fat, if preferred)
- 2 tablespoons Sriracha sauce
- 1 tablespoon lime juice
- 1 clove garlic, minced

Preparation:

1. In a small bowl, combine mayonnaise, Sriracha sauce, lime juice, and minced garlic.
2. Stir well to combine.
3. Taste and adjust seasoning if necessary, adding more Sriracha for extra heat if desired.
4. Serve immediately as a dip for fries, a sauce for sandwiches or wraps, or as a topping for burgers or tacos.

Nutrient Facts (per serving):

- Calories: 80
- Carbohydrates: 1g
- Fat: 9g
- Protein: 0g

12. Avocado Lime Crema

Prep.Time: 5 min | **Cook Time:** 0 min | **Serving:** 4

Ingredients:

- 1 ripe avocado
- 1/4 cup Greek yogurt (low-fat or non-fat)
- 2 tablespoons lime juice
- 1 clove garlic, minced
- Salt and pepper to taste

Preparation:

1. In a food processor or blender, combine ripe avocado, Greek yogurt, lime juice, and minced garlic.
2. Blend until smooth and creamy.
3. Season with salt and pepper according to taste.
4. Taste and adjust seasoning if necessary.
5. Serve immediately as a topping for tacos, grilled fish, salads, or as a dip for vegetable sticks or tortilla chips.

Nutrient Facts (per serving):

- Calories: 60
- Carbohydrates: 3g
- Fat: 5g
- Protein: 1g

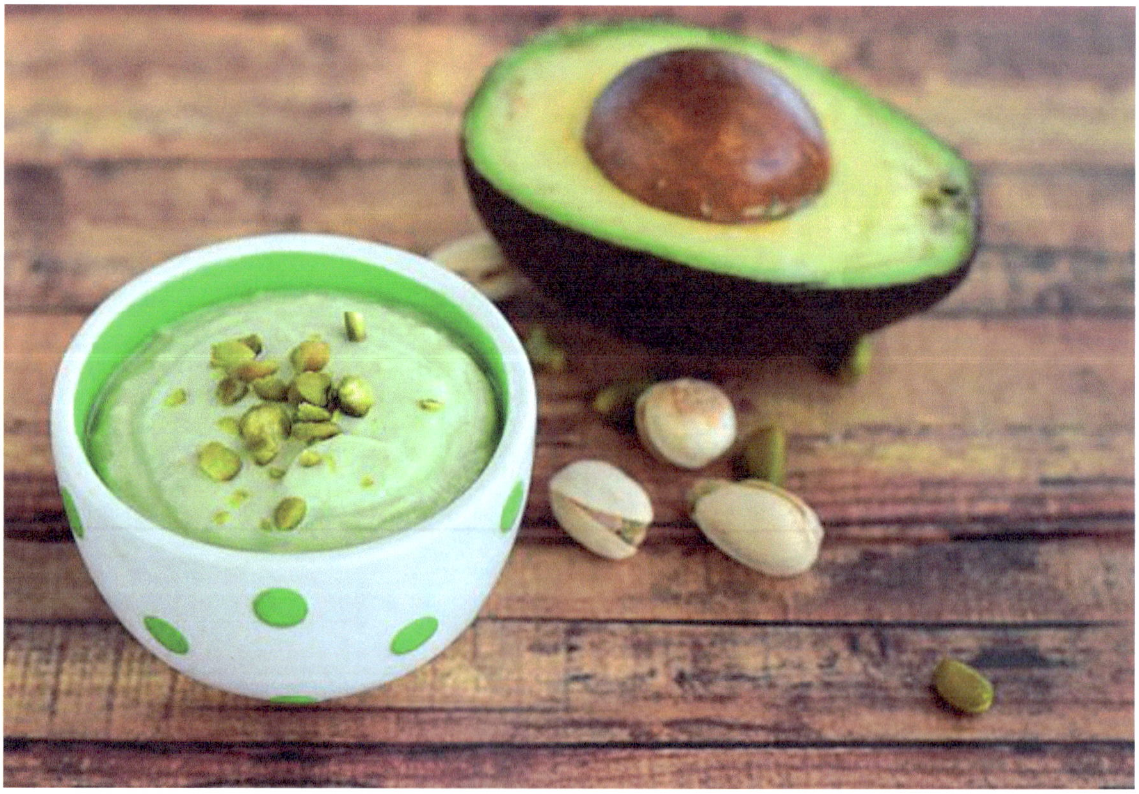

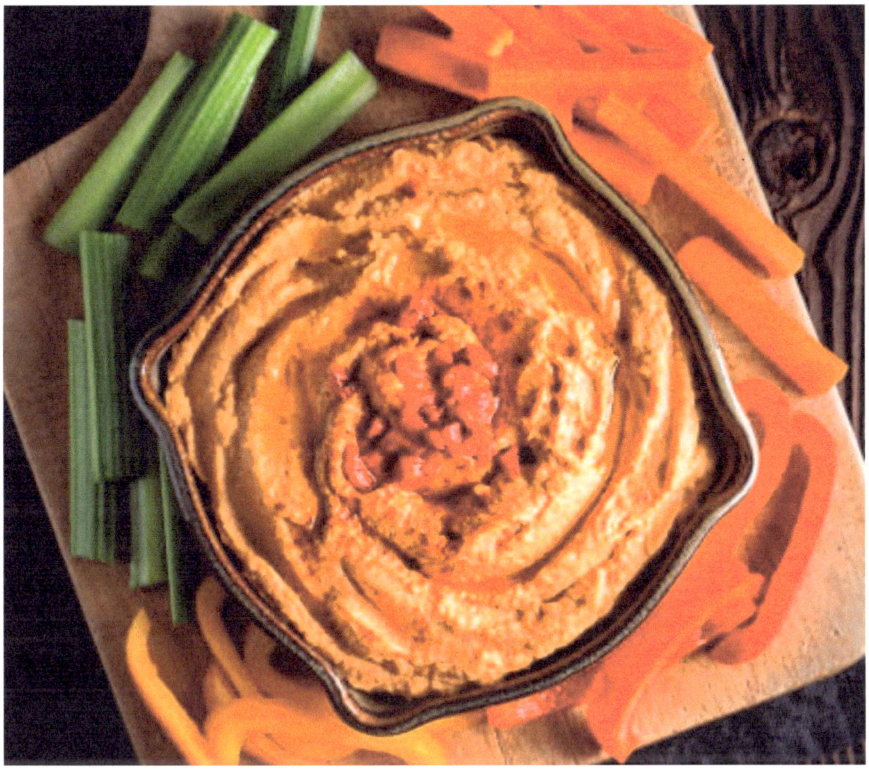

13. Roasted Red Pepper Hummus

Prep.Time: 15 min | **Cook Time:** 25 min | **Serving:** 4

Ingredients:

- 1 can (15 ounces) chickpeas (garbanzo beans), drained and rinsed
- 1 roasted red pepper, peeled and seeded
- 2 tablespoons tahini (sesame seed paste)
- 2 cloves garlic, minced
- 2 tablespoons lemon juice
- 2 tablespoons extra virgin olive oil
- Salt and pepper to taste

Preparation:

1. Preheat the oven to 425°F (220°C).
2. Place the red pepper on a baking sheet and roast in the preheated oven for 20-25 minutes, until charred and softened.
3. Remove the red pepper from the oven and let cool slightly before peeling off the skin and removing the seeds.
4. In a food processor, combine chickpeas, roasted red pepper, tahini, minced garlic, lemon juice, and olive oil.
5. Blend until smooth, scraping down the sides of the processor as needed.
6. If the hummus is too thick, add water, 1 tablespoon at a time, until desired consistency is reached.
7. Season with salt and pepper according to taste.
8. Transfer the hummus to a serving bowl.
9. Drizzle with a little extra olive oil, if desired.
10. Serve with vegetable sticks, whole grain pita bread, or as a spread for sandwiches or wraps.

Nutrient Facts (per serving):

- Calories: 70
- Carbohydrates: 8g
- Fat: 3g
- Protein: 3g

14. Garlic Parmesan Dressing

Prep.Time: 5 min | **Cook Time:** 0 min | **Serving:** 4

Ingredients:

- 1/4 cup grated Parmesan cheese
- 1/4 cup mayonnaise (light or low-fat, if preferred)
- 2 tablespoons extra virgin olive oil
- 1 tablespoon lemon juice
- 1 clove garlic, minced
- Salt and pepper to taste

Preparation:

1. In a small bowl, whisk together grated Parmesan cheese, mayonnaise, extra virgin olive oil, lemon juice, and minced garlic until well combined.
2. Season with salt and pepper according to taste.
3. Taste and adjust seasoning if necessary.
4. Serve immediately over salads or as a dip for vegetables.

Nutrient Facts (per serving):

- Calories: 90
- Carbohydrates: 2g
- Fat: 8g
- Protein: 2g

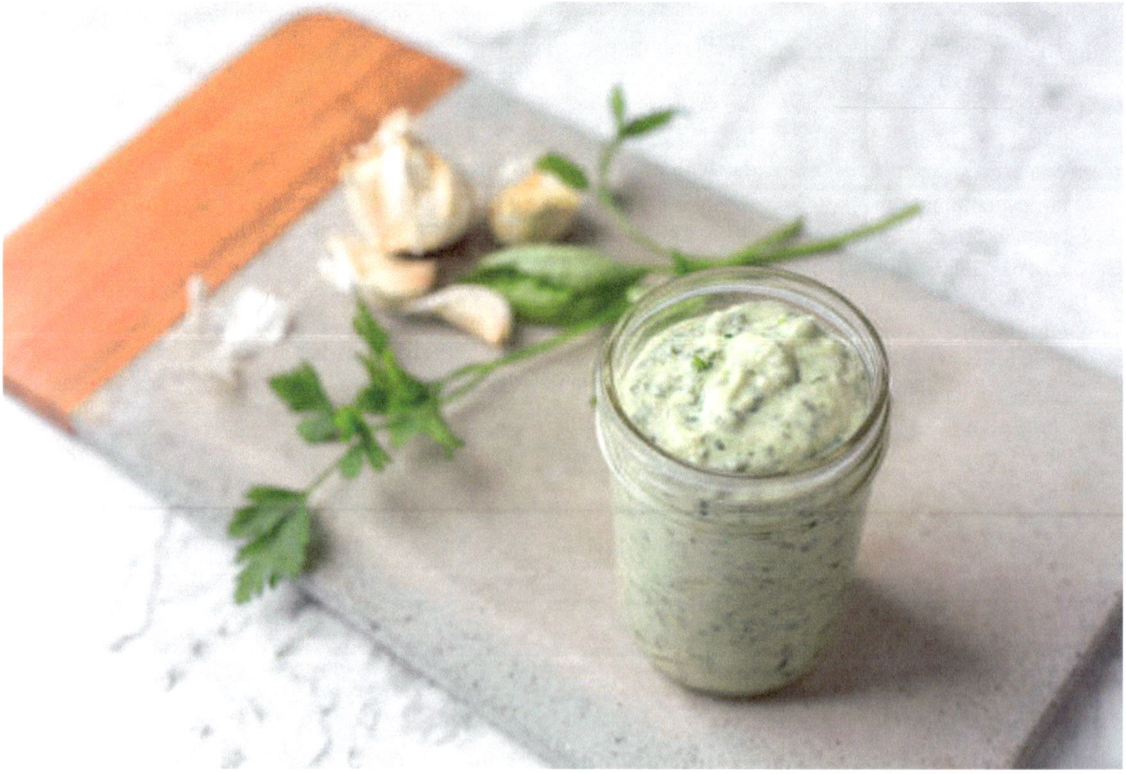

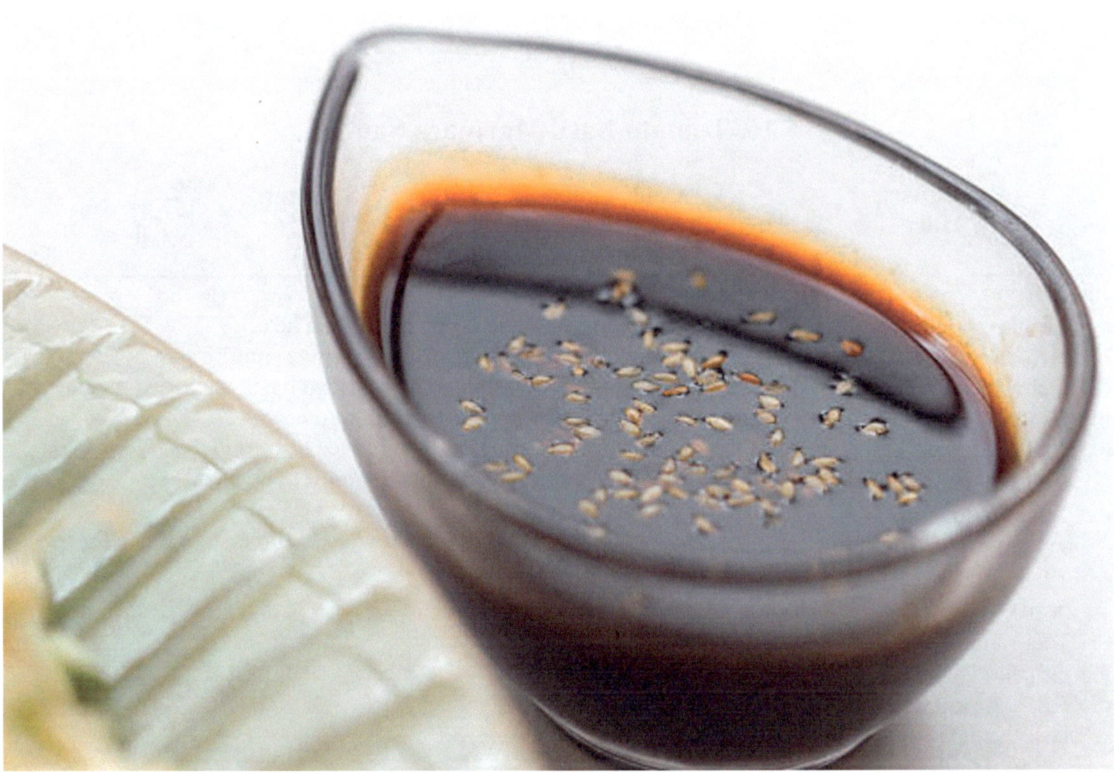

15. Soy Ginger Dipping Sauce

Prep.Time: 5 min

Cook Time: 0 min

Serving: 4

Ingredients:

- 3 tablespoons low-sodium soy sauce
- 1 tablespoon rice vinegar
- 1 tablespoon honey or maple syrup
- 1 teaspoon grated fresh ginger
- 1 clove garlic, minced
- 1 green onion, thinly sliced (optional)

Preparation:

1. In a small bowl, whisk together soy sauce, rice vinegar, honey or maple syrup, grated ginger, and minced garlic until well combined.
2. Stir in sliced green onion, if using.
3. Taste and adjust seasoning if necessary.
4. Serve immediately as a dipping sauce for sushi, spring rolls, dumplings, or grilled meats and vegetables.

Nutrient Facts (per serving):

- Calories: 40
- Carbohydrates: 5g
- Fat: 2g
- Protein: 1g

16. Tomato Basil Marinara Sauce

Prep.Time: 10 min

Cook Time: 25 min

Serving: 4

Ingredients:

- 2 tablespoons olive oil
- 2 cloves garlic, minced
- 1 can (14 ounces) diced tomatoes
- 1 can (6 ounces) tomato paste
- 1 teaspoon dried basil
- 1 teaspoon dried oregano
- Salt and pepper to taste

Preparation:

1. In a saucepan, heat olive oil over medium heat.
2. Add minced garlic and sauté for 1-2 minutes until fragrant.
3. Stir in diced tomatoes, tomato paste, dried basil, and dried oregano.
4. Season with salt and pepper according to taste.
5. Bring the sauce to a simmer, then reduce heat to low and let it cook for about 20-25 minutes, stirring occasionally, until thickened.
6. Taste and adjust seasoning if necessary.
7. Serve over cooked pasta, spaghetti squash, or use as a sauce for pizza or dipping breadsticks.

Nutrient Facts (per serving):

- Calories: 50
- Carbohydrates: 7g
- Fat: 2g
- Protein: 1g

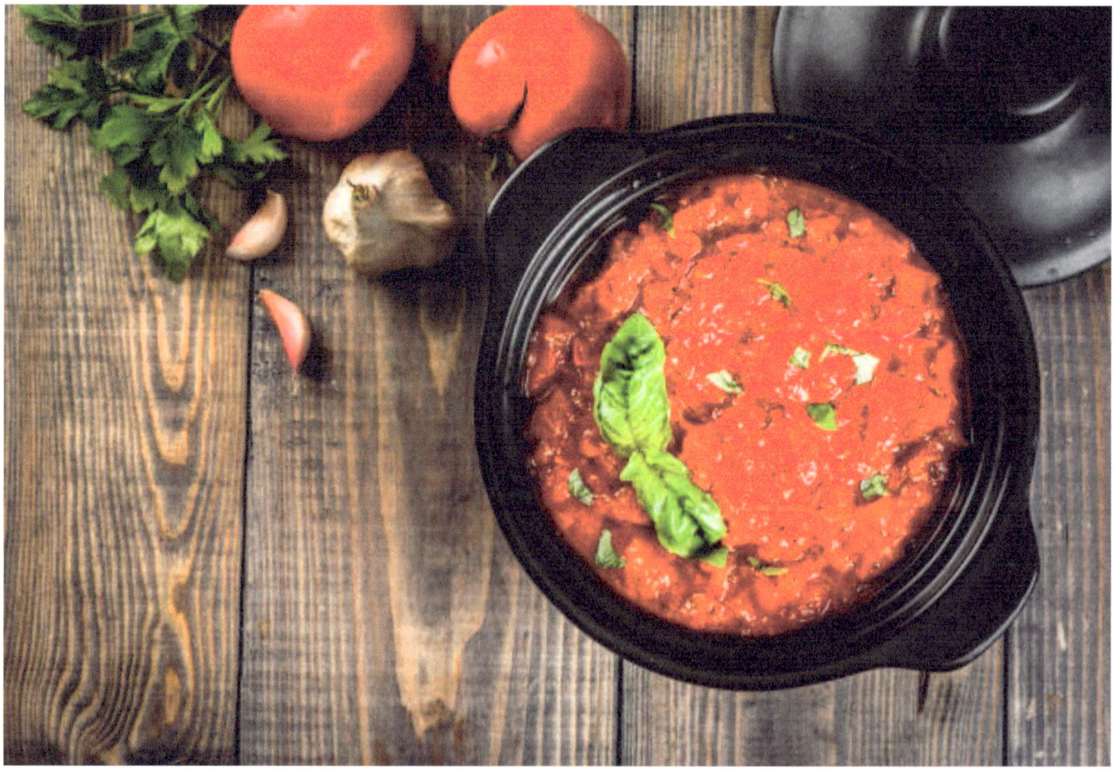

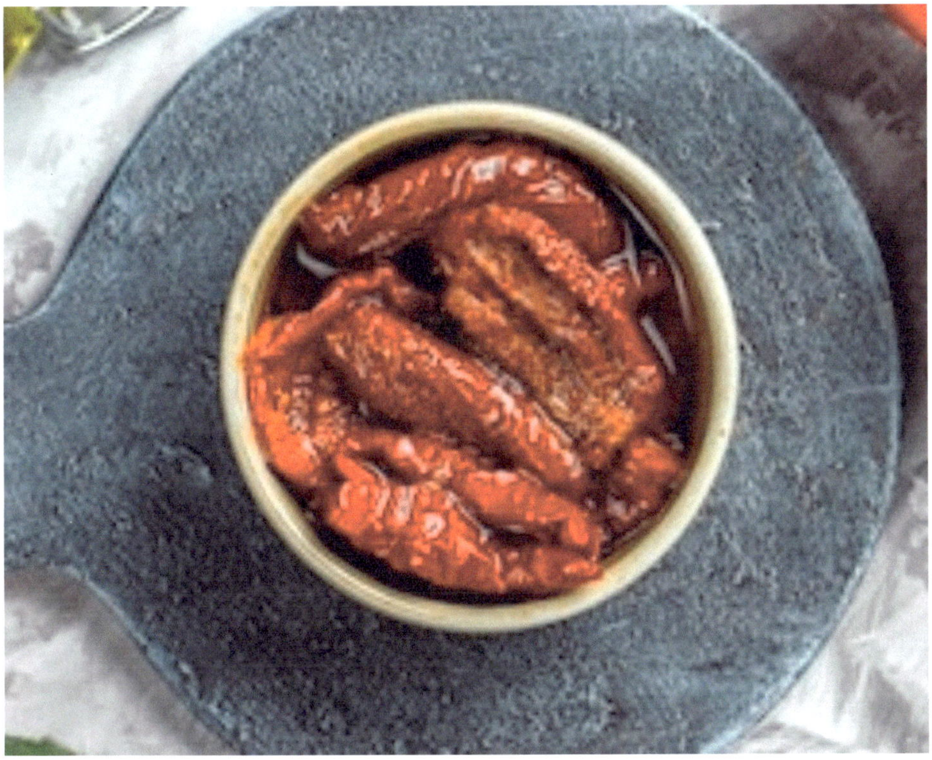

17. Walnut and Roasted Red Pepper Pesto

Prep.Time: 10 min | **Cook Time:** 0 min | **Serving:** 4

Ingredients:

- 1 cup packed fresh basil leaves
- 1/4 cup walnuts
- 1/4 cup grated Parmesan cheese
- 1/4 cup roasted red peppers, drained
- 1 clove garlic, minced
- 2 tablespoons extra virgin olive oil
- Salt and pepper to taste

Preparation:

1. In a food processor, combine basil leaves, walnuts, grated Parmesan cheese, roasted red peppers, and minced garlic.
2. Pulse until coarsely chopped.
3. While the food processor is running, gradually add the olive oil in a steady stream until the pesto reaches your desired consistency.
4. Season with salt and pepper according to taste.
5. Taste and adjust seasoning if necessary.
6. Transfer the pesto to a serving bowl.
7. Serve with cooked pasta, spread on sandwiches or wraps, or use as a topping for grilled meats or fish.

Nutrient Facts (per serving):

- Calories: 120
- Carbohydrates: 4g
- Fat: 11g
- Protein: 3g

18. Buffalo Cauliflower Dip

Prep.Time: 15 min | **Cook Time:** 25 min | **Serving:** 4

Ingredients:

- 1 small head cauliflower, cut into florets
- 2 tablespoons olive oil
- Salt and pepper to taste
- 1/4 cup buffalo sauce (check for sugar-free version)
- 1/4 cup Greek yogurt (low-fat or non-fat)
- 2 tablespoons mayonnaise (light or low-fat, if preferred)
- 1 tablespoon lemon juice
- 1 clove garlic, minced
- 2 green onions, thinly sliced
- Celery sticks and carrot sticks, for serving

Preparation:

1. Preheat the oven to 425°F (220°C).
2. Place cauliflower florets on a baking sheet.
3. Drizzle with olive oil and season with salt and pepper.
4. Toss to coat evenly.
5. Roast in the preheated oven for 20-25 minutes, until cauliflower is tender and lightly browned.
6. In a small bowl, whisk together buffalo sauce, Greek yogurt, mayonnaise, lemon juice, and minced garlic until well combined.
7. Once the cauliflower is done, transfer it to a serving dish.
8. Pour the buffalo sauce mixture over the roasted cauliflower and gently toss to coat.
9. Garnish with sliced green onions.
10. Serve warm with celery sticks and carrot sticks for dipping.

Nutrient Facts (per serving):

- Calories: 60
- Carbohydrates: 5g
- Fat: 4g
- Protein: 2g

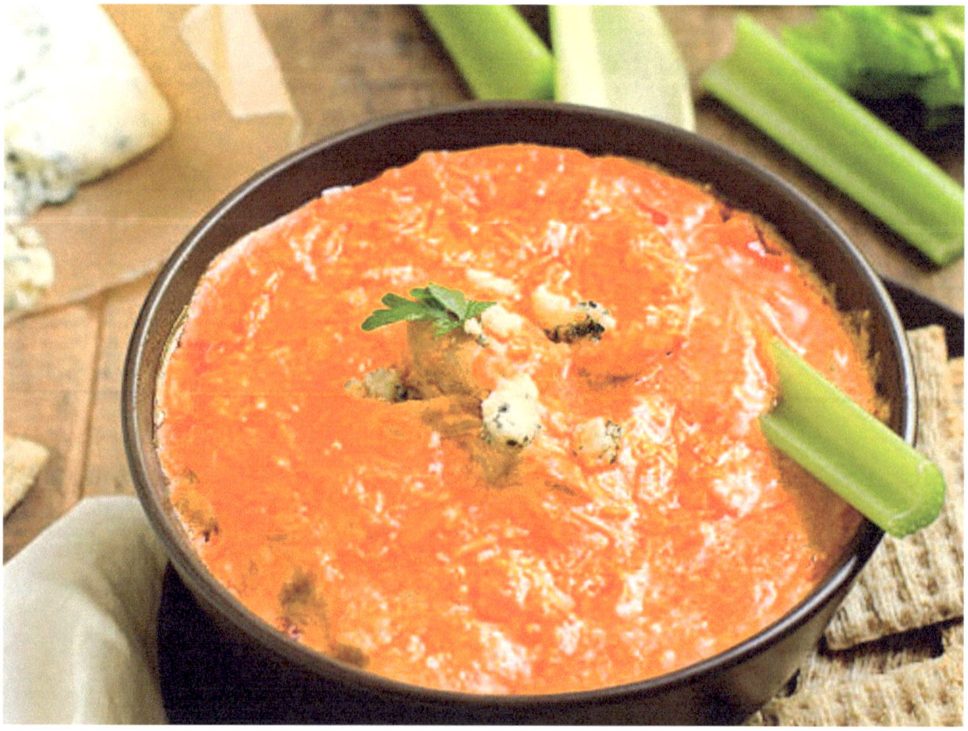

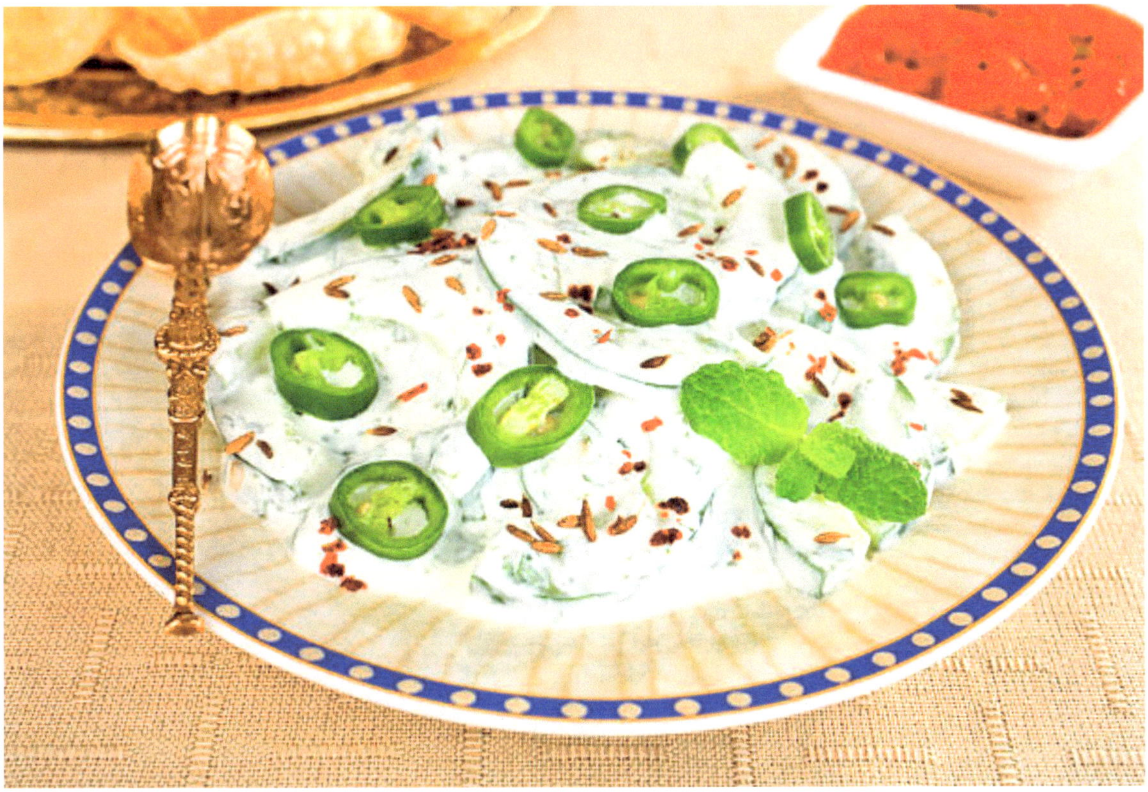

19. Chipotle Lime Greek Yogurt Sauce

Prep.Time: 5 min

Cook Time: 0 min

Serving: 4

Ingredients:

- 1/2 cup Greek yogurt (low-fat or non-fat)
- 1 chipotle pepper in adobo sauce, minced
- 1 tablespoon lime juice
- 1 clove garlic, minced
- Salt to taste
- Add chipotle or Jalapeno Peppers to taste

Preparation:

1. In a small bowl, combine Greek yogurt, minced chipotle pepper, lime juice, and minced garlic.
2. Stir well to combine.
3. Season with salt according to taste.
4. Taste and adjust seasoning if necessary.
5. Serve immediately as a dipping sauce for grilled meats, vegetables, or as a topping for tacos or salads.

Nutrient Facts (per serving):

- Calories: 50
- Carbohydrates: 3g
- Fat: 3g
- Protein: 3g

20. Mango Salsa with Jalapeño

Prep.Time:	Cook Time:	Serving:
10 min	0 min	4

Ingredients:

- 1 ripe mango, peeled, pitted, and diced
- 1/4 cup diced red onion
- 1 jalapeño pepper, seeded and finely chopped
- 1/4 cup chopped fresh cilantro
- 1 tablespoon lime juice
- Salt to taste

Preparation:

1. In a mixing bowl, combine diced mango, diced red onion, chopped jalapeño pepper, chopped cilantro, and lime juice.
2. Stir well to combine.
3. Season with salt according to taste.
4. Taste and adjust seasoning if necessary.
5. Serve immediately as a topping for grilled fish or chicken, or as a dip with tortilla chips.

Nutrient Facts (per serving):

- Calories: 40
- Carbohydrates: 10g
- Fat: 0g
- Protein: 1g

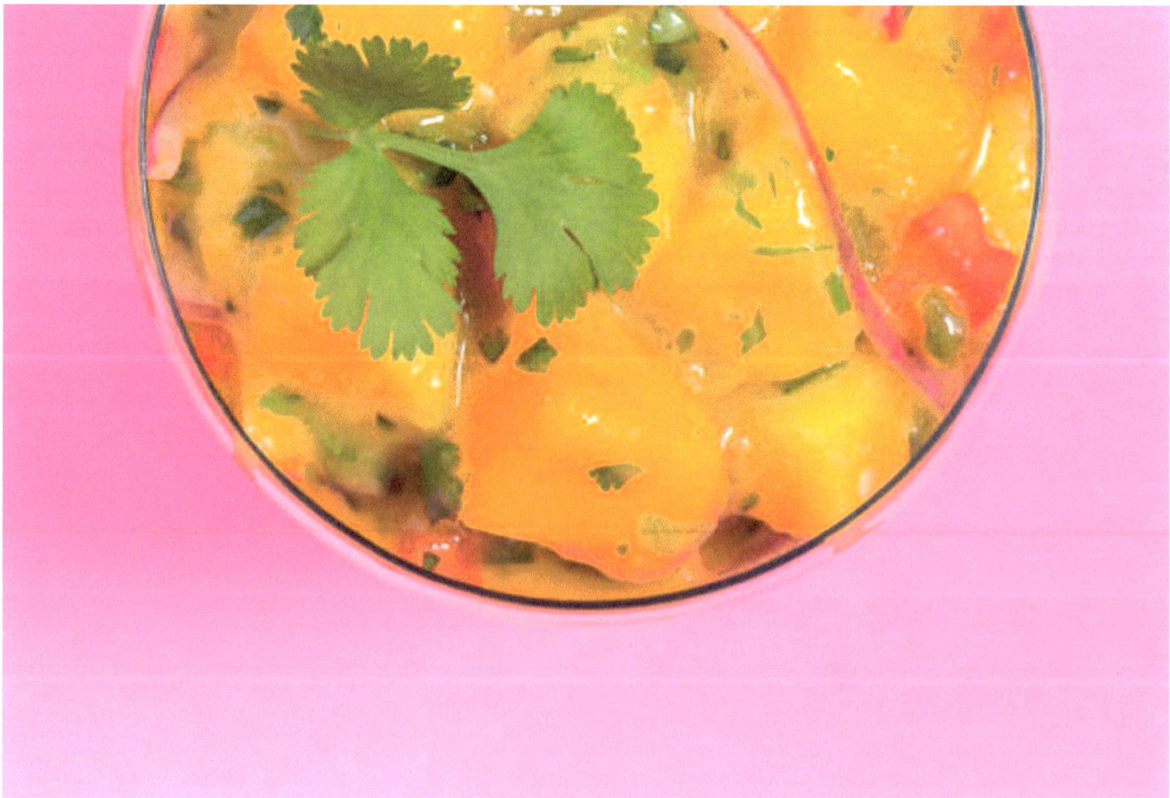

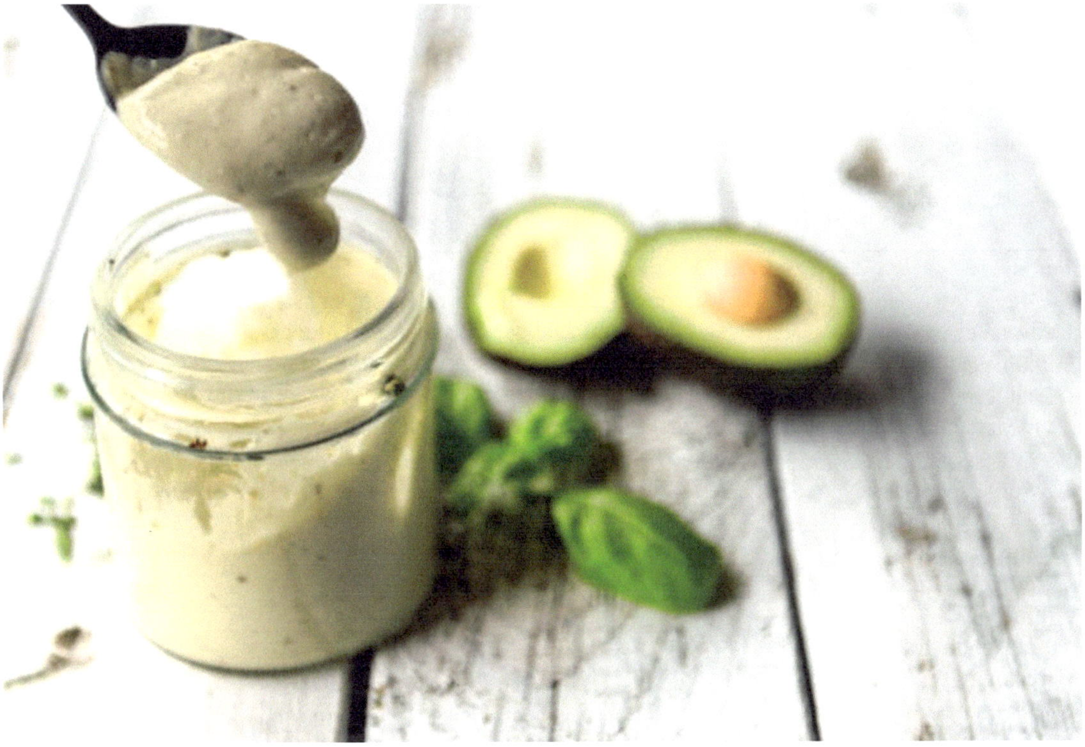

21. Cilantro Lime Avocado Dressing

Prep.Time: 5 min

Cook Time: 0 min

Serving: 4

Ingredients:

- 1 ripe avocado
- 1/4 cup Greek yogurt (low-fat or non-fat)
- 2 tablespoons lime juice
- 2 tablespoons chopped fresh cilantro
- 1 clove garlic, minced
- Salt and pepper to taste

Preparation:

1. In a food processor or blender, combine ripe avocado, Greek yogurt, lime juice, chopped cilantro, and minced garlic.
2. Blend until smooth and creamy.
3. Season with salt and pepper according to taste.
4. Taste and adjust seasoning if necessary.
5. Serve immediately over salads, grilled vegetables, or as a dip for vegetable sticks or tortilla chips.

Nutrient Facts (per serving):

- Calories: 90
- Carbohydrates: 5g
- Fat: 8g
- Protein: 1g

22. Sugar-Free Teriyaki Sauce

Prep.Time: 5 min | **Cook Time:** 10 min | **Serving:** 4

Ingredients:

- 1/4 cup low-sodium soy sauce
- 2 tablespoons water
- 2 tablespoons rice vinegar
- 2 tablespoons Swerve sweetener (or any other sugar-free sweetener)
- 1 clove garlic, minced
- 1 teaspoon grated fresh ginger
- 1 teaspoon cornstarch (mixed with 1 tablespoon water)

Preparation:

1. In a saucepan, combine low-sodium soy sauce, water, rice vinegar, Swerve sweetener, minced garlic, and grated ginger.
2. Bring the mixture to a simmer over medium heat.
3. In a small bowl, mix cornstarch with water until dissolved to create a slurry.
4. Gradually add the cornstarch slurry to the saucepan, stirring constantly, until the sauce thickens to your desired consistency.
5. Remove from heat and let cool slightly before serving.
6. Taste and adjust seasoning if necessary.
7. Serve as a marinade for grilled chicken, tofu, or vegetables, or as a dipping sauce for sushi or spring rolls.

Nutrient Facts (per serving):

- Calories: 30
- Carbohydrates: 5g
- Fat: 0g
- Protein: 2g

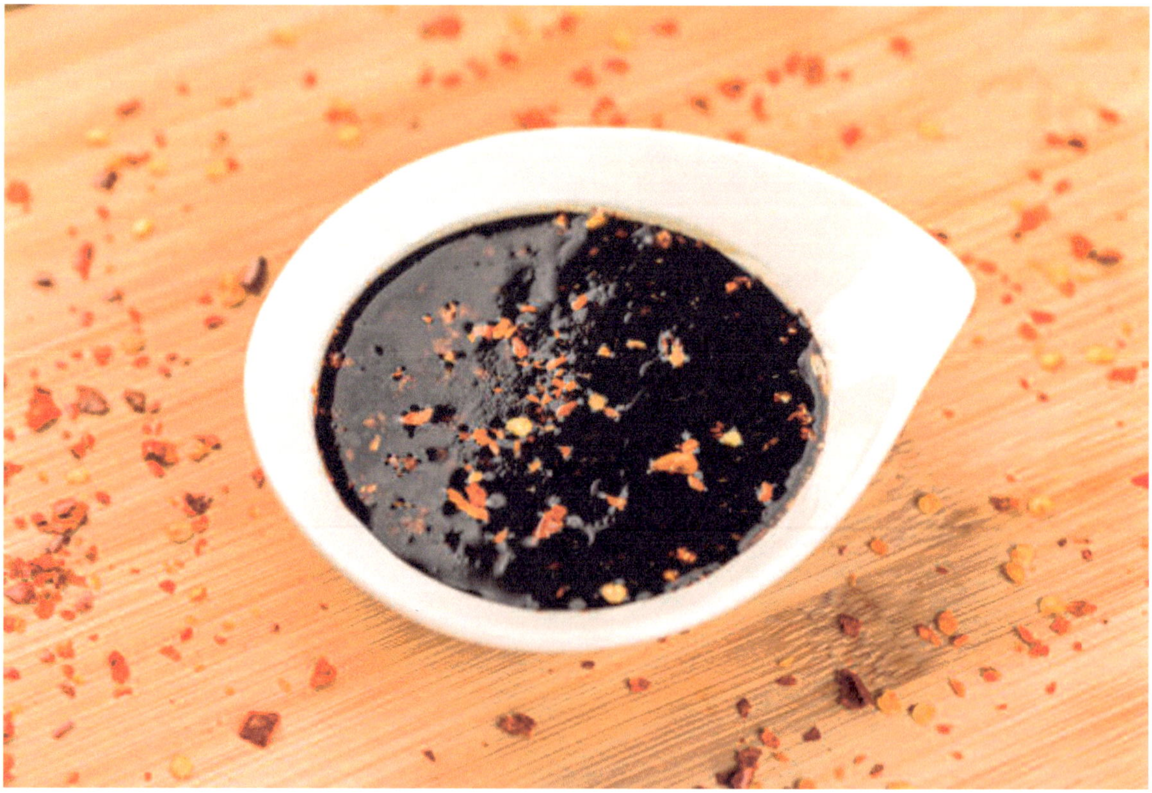

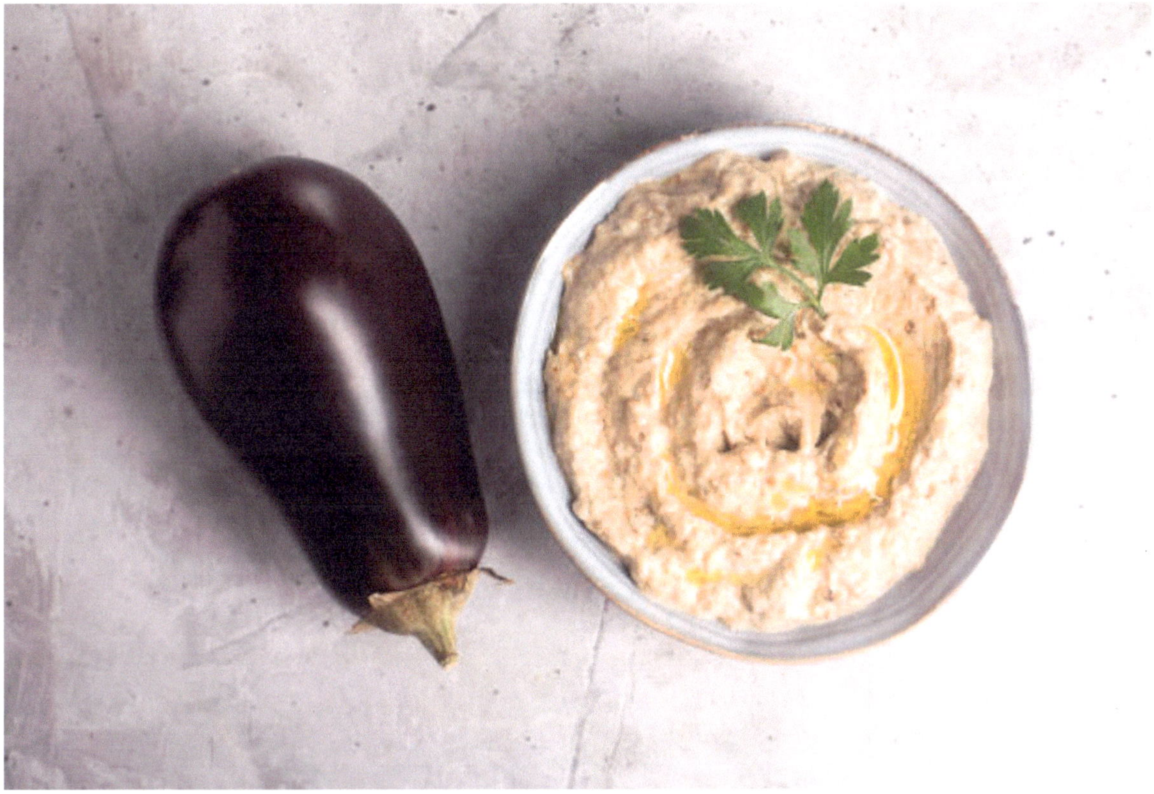

23. Roasted Eggplant Baba Ganoush

Prep.Time: 15 min

Cook Time: 40 min

Serving: 4

Ingredients:

- 1 large eggplant
- 2 cloves garlic, minced
- 2 tablespoons tahini (sesame seed paste)
- 2 tablespoons lemon juice
- 1 tablespoon extra virgin olive oil
- 1/2 teaspoon ground cumin
- Salt and pepper to taste
- Chopped fresh parsley for garnish

Preparation:

1. Preheat the oven to 400°F (200°C).
2. Prick the eggplant with a fork in several places and place it on a baking sheet.
3. Roast the eggplant in the preheated oven for 40-45 minutes, or until the skin is charred and the flesh is soft.
4. Remove the eggplant from the oven and let it cool slightly.
5. Cut the eggplant in half and scoop out the flesh into a food processor.
6. Add minced garlic, tahini, lemon juice, olive oil, ground cumin, salt, and pepper.
7. Blend until smooth and creamy.
8. Taste and adjust seasoning if necessary.
9. Transfer the baba ganoush to a serving bowl, drizzle with a little extra olive oil, and garnish with chopped fresh parsley.
10. Serve with pita bread, crackers, or vegetable sticks.

Nutrient Facts (per serving):

- Calories: 70
- Carbohydrates: 6g
- Fat: 5g
- Protein: 1g

24. Lemon Herb Vinaigrette

Prep.Time:	Cook Time:	Serving:
5 min	0 min	4

Ingredients:

- 1/4 cup extra virgin olive oil
- 2 tablespoons lemon juice
- 1 tablespoon chopped fresh herbs (such as basil, parsley, or thyme)
- 1 teaspoon Dijon mustard
- 1 clove garlic, minced
- Salt and pepper to taste

Preparation:

1. In a small bowl, whisk together extra virgin olive oil, lemon juice, chopped fresh herbs, Dijon mustard, and minced garlic until well combined.
2. Season with salt and pepper according to taste.
3. Taste and adjust seasoning if necessary.
4. Serve immediately over salads or grilled vegetables.

Nutrient Facts (per serving):

- Calories: 60
- Carbohydrates: 2g
- Fat: 6g
- Protein: 0g

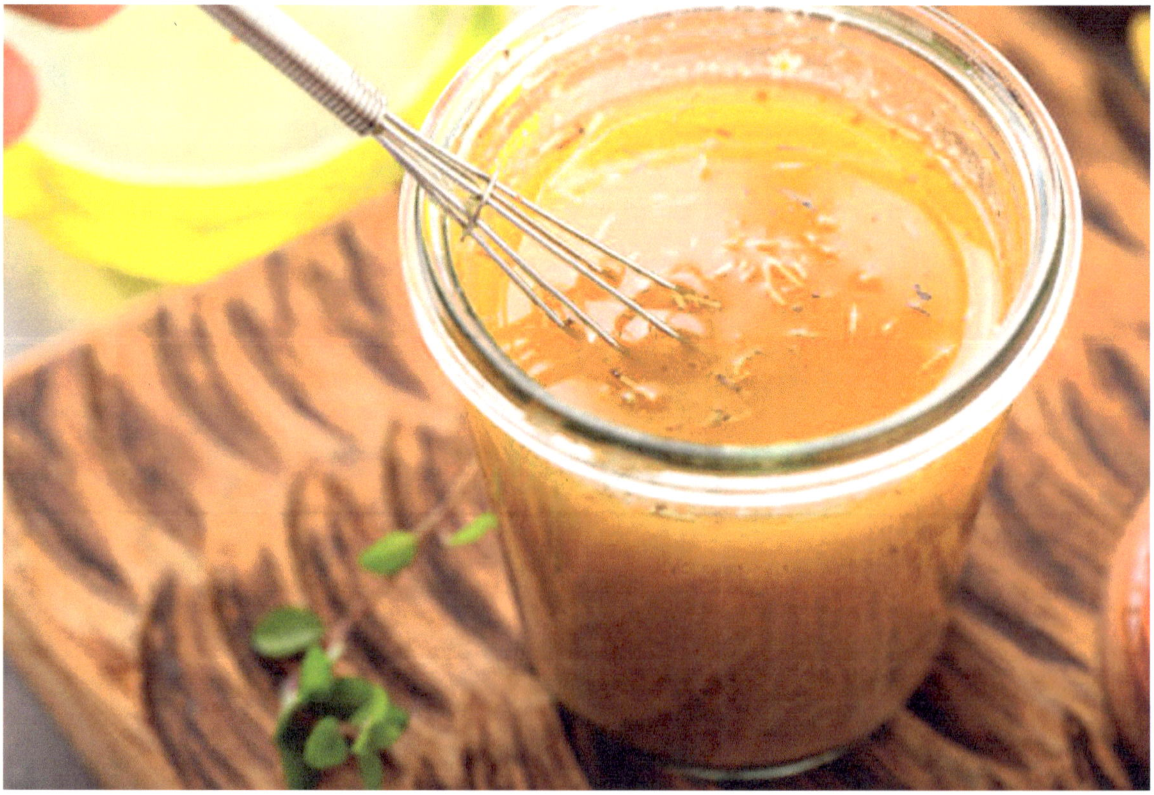

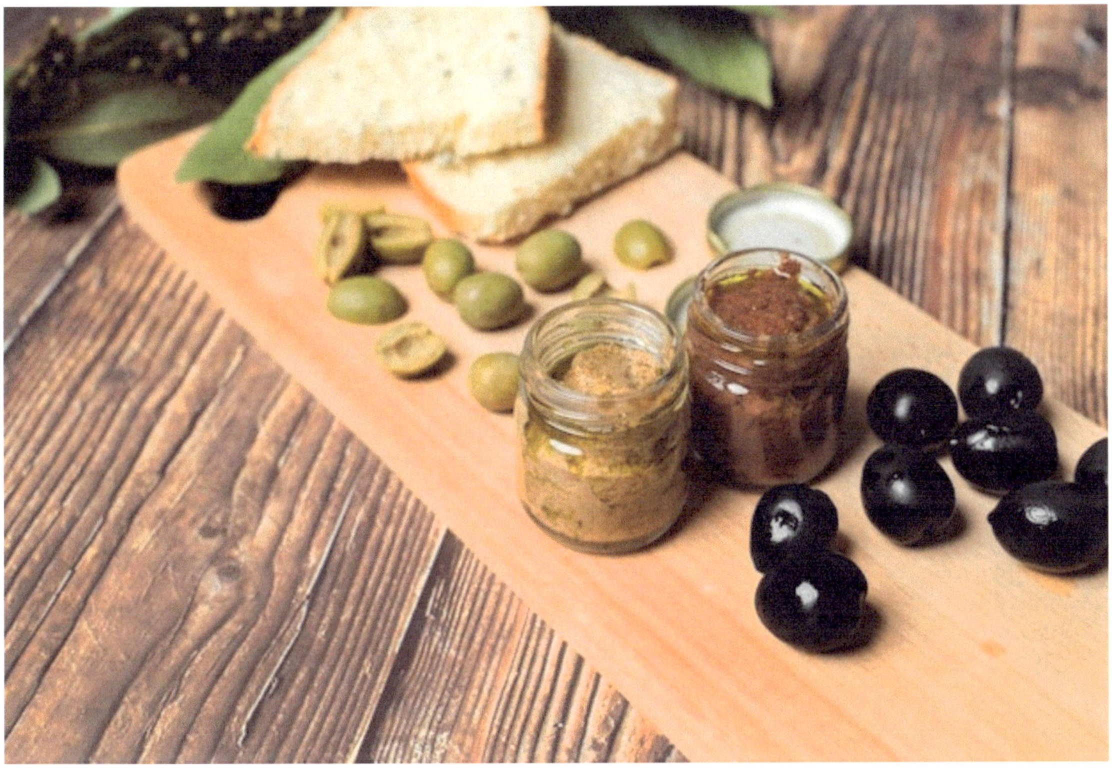

25. Greek Olive Tapenade

Prep.Time: 10 min

Cook Time: 0 min

Serving: 4

Ingredients:

- 1 cup mixed Greek olives, pitted
- 2 tablespoons capers
- 2 cloves garlic, minced
- 1 tablespoon chopped fresh parsley
- 1 tablespoon lemon juice
- 2 tablespoons extra virgin olive oil
- Freshly ground black pepper to taste

Preparation:

1. In a food processor, combine Greek olives, capers, minced garlic, chopped parsley, lemon juice, and extra virgin olive oil.
2. Pulse until the mixture is finely chopped and reaches your desired consistency.
3. Season with freshly ground black pepper according to taste.
4. Taste and adjust seasoning if necessary.
5. Transfer the tapenade to a serving bowl.
6. Serve with crackers, toasted bread, or as a topping for grilled fish or chicken.

Nutrient Facts (per serving):

- Calories: 80
- Carbohydrates: 2g
- Fat: 8g
- Protein: 1g

26. Low-Sodium Dill Pickle Dip

Prep.Time: 5 min | **Cook Time:** 0 min | **Serving:** 4

Ingredients:

- 1/2 cup Greek yogurt (low-fat or non-fat)
- 1/4 cup finely chopped dill pickles
- 1 tablespoon pickle juice
- 1 clove garlic, minced
- 1 teaspoon dried dill
- Salt and pepper to taste
- Add cilantro or spinach to taste

Preparation:

1. In a small bowl, combine Greek yogurt, chopped dill pickles, pickle juice, minced garlic, and dried dill.
2. Stir well to combine.
3. Season with salt and pepper according to taste.
4. Taste and adjust seasoning if necessary.
5. Serve immediately with potato chips, pretzels, or vegetable sticks.

Nutrient Facts (per serving):

- Calories: 40
- Carbohydrates: 2g
- Fat: 3g
- Protein: 1g

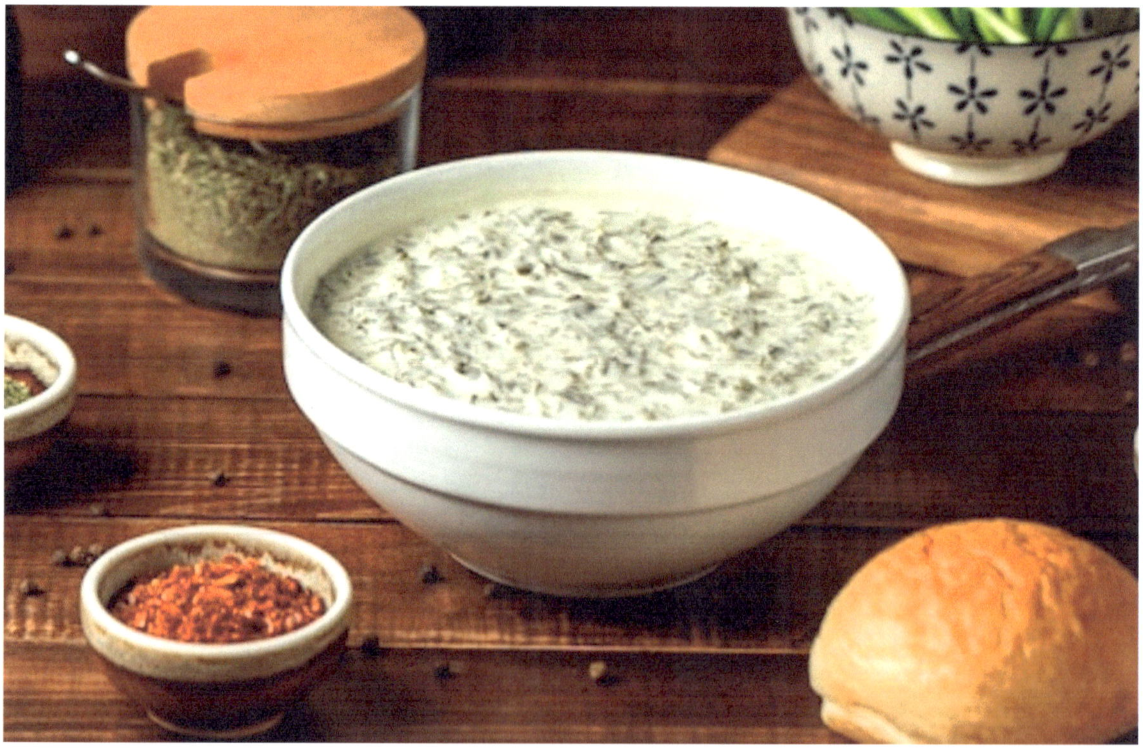

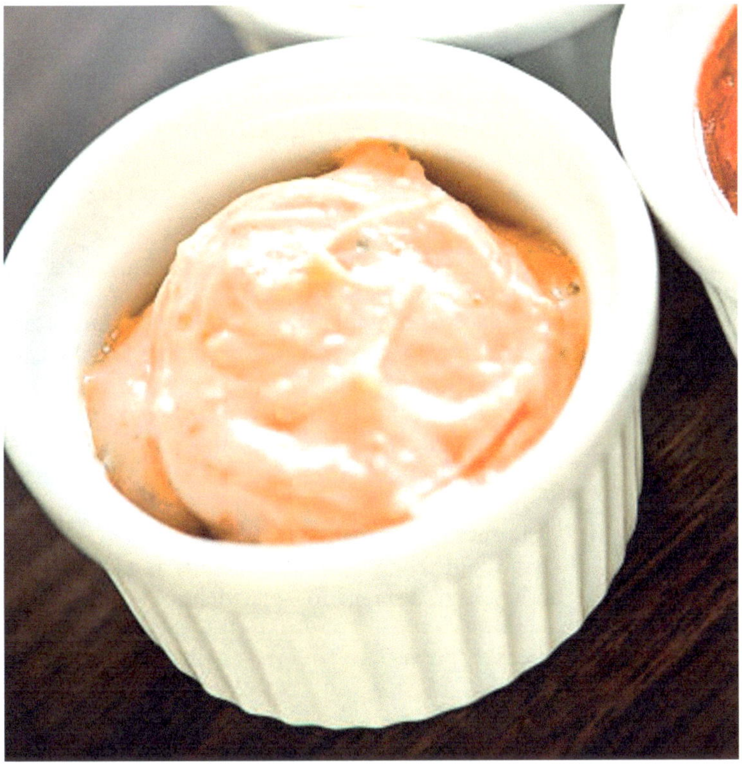

27. Cajun Remoulade Sauce

Prep.Time: 10 min | **Cook Time:** 0 min | **Serving:** 4

Ingredients:

- 1/2 cup mayonnaise
- 2 tablespoons Creole mustard
- 1 tablespoon chopped fresh parsley
- 1 tablespoon chopped green onions
- 1 tablespoon lemon juice
- 1 teaspoon Worcestershire sauce
- 1 clove garlic, minced
- 1/2 teaspoon paprika
- 1/2 teaspoon Cajun seasoning
- Salt and pepper to taste

Preparation:

1. In a small bowl, combine mayonnaise, Creole mustard, chopped parsley, chopped green onions, lemon juice, Worcestershire sauce, minced garlic, paprika, and Cajun seasoning.
2. Stir well to combine.
3. Season with salt and pepper according to taste.
4. Taste and adjust seasoning if necessary.
5. Serve immediately as a dipping sauce for seafood, as a spread for sandwiches, or as a dressing for salads.

Nutrient Facts (per serving):

- Calories: 70
- Carbohydrates: 2g
- Fat: 7g
- Protein: 1g

28. Cranberry Orange Chutney

Prep.Time: 5 min | **Cook Time:** 20 min | **Serving:** 4

Ingredients:

- 1 cup fresh cranberries
- 1 orange, zest and juice
- 1/4 cup honey or maple syrup
- 1/4 cup water
- 1/2 teaspoon ground cinnamon
- 1/4 teaspoon ground ginger
- Pinch of salt

Preparation:

1. In a saucepan, combine fresh cranberries, orange zest, orange juice, honey or maple syrup, water, ground cinnamon, ground ginger, and a pinch of salt.
2. Stir well to combine.
3. Bring the mixture to a boil over medium heat.
4. Reduce heat to low and let it simmer for about 15-20 minutes, stirring occasionally, until the cranberries burst and the mixture thickens.
5. Remove from heat and let cool before serving.
6. Transfer to a serving dish.
7. Serve chilled or at room temperature as a condiment for roasted meats, turkey, or as a spread for sandwiches.

Nutrient Facts (per serving):

- Calories: 70
- Carbohydrates: 18g
- Fat: 0g
- Protein: 0g

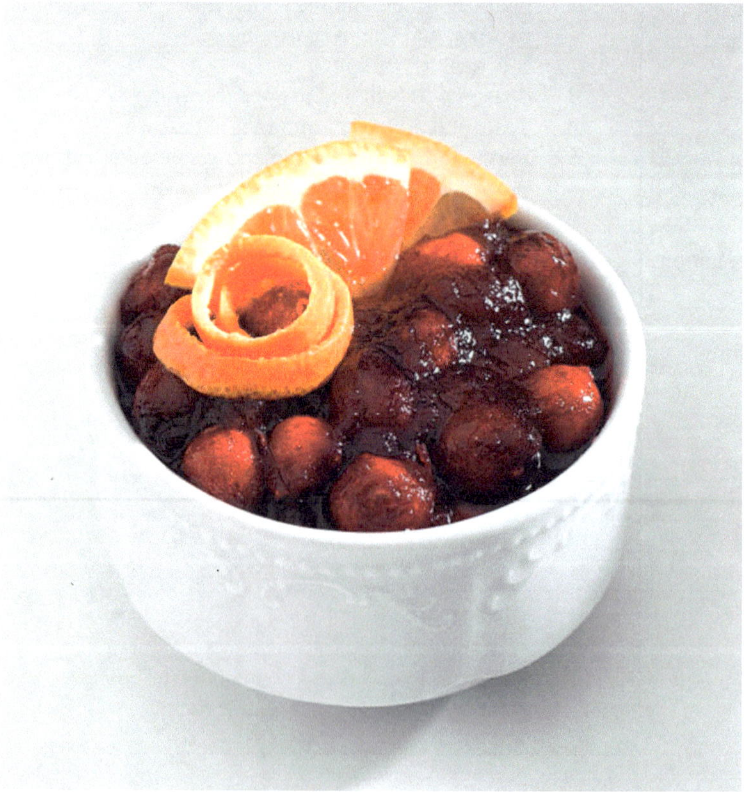

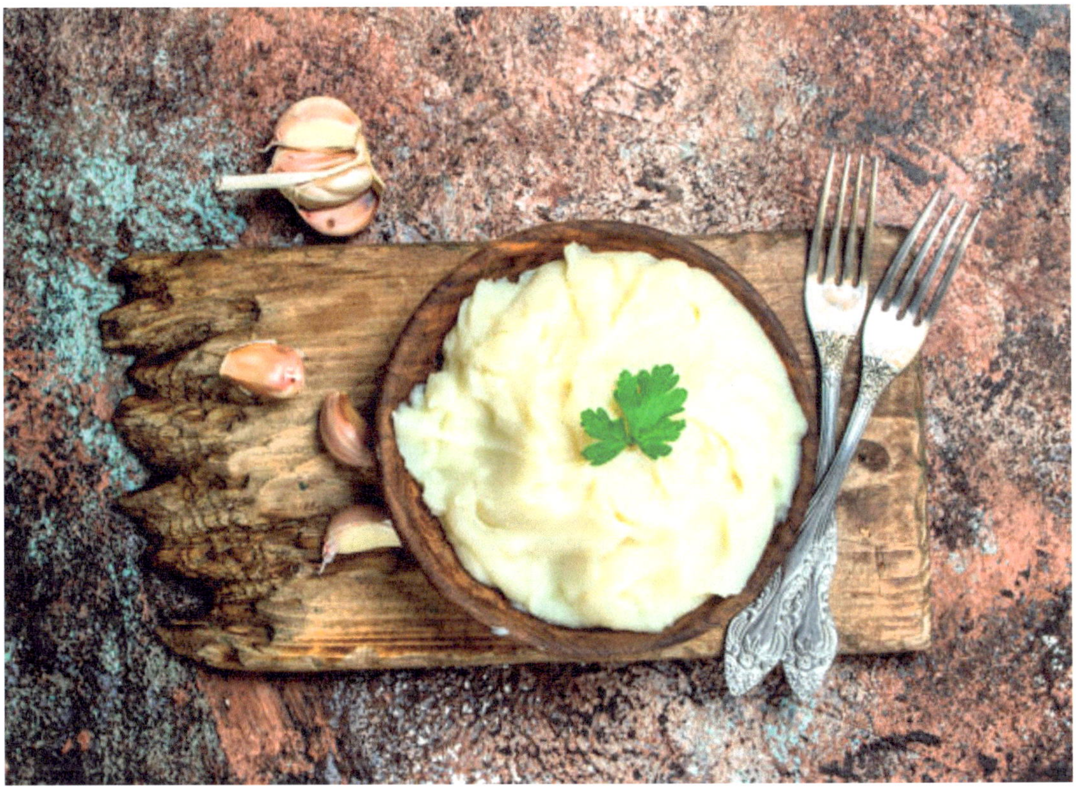

29. Roasted Garlic Aioli

Prep.Time:	Cook Time:	Serving:
5 min	25 min	4

Ingredients:

- 1 head garlic
- 1/4 cup mayonnaise (light or low-fat, if preferred)
- 1 tablespoon lemon juice
- Salt and pepper to taste

Preparation:

1. Preheat the oven to 400°F (200°C).
2. Slice off the top of the garlic head to expose the cloves.
3. Place the garlic head on a piece of aluminum foil and drizzle with a little olive oil.
4. Wrap the garlic in the foil and place it on a baking sheet.
5. Roast in the preheated oven for 25-30 minutes, or until the garlic cloves are soft and golden brown.
6. Remove from the oven and let cool slightly.
7. Squeeze the roasted garlic cloves out of their skins into a small bowl.
8. Mash the roasted garlic cloves with a fork until smooth.
9. Add mayonnaise and lemon juice to the mashed garlic.
10. Stir well to combine.
11. Season with salt and pepper according to taste.
12. Taste and adjust seasoning if necessary.
13. Transfer to a serving bowl.
14. Serve as a dipping sauce for fries, roasted vegetables, or as a spread for sandwiches or burgers.

Nutrient Facts (per serving):

- Calories: 90
- Carbohydrates: 1g
- Fat: 10g
- Protein: 0g

30. Pumpkin Seed and Cilantro Pesto

Prep.Time: 10 min | **Cook Time:** 0 min | **Serving:** 4

Ingredients:

- 1 cup fresh cilantro leaves
- 1/4 cup pumpkin seeds (pepitas)
- 1/4 cup grated Parmesan cheese
- 1 clove garlic, minced
- 2 tablespoons lemon juice
- 1/4 cup extra virgin olive oil
- Salt and pepper to taste

Preparation:

1. In a food processor, combine cilantro leaves, pumpkin seeds, grated Parmesan cheese, minced garlic, and lemon juice.
2. Pulse until coarsely chopped.
3. While the food processor is running, gradually add the olive oil in a steady stream until the pesto reaches your desired consistency.
4. Season with salt and pepper according to taste.
5. Taste and adjust seasoning if necessary.
6. Transfer the pesto to a serving bowl.
7. Serve with cooked pasta, spread on sandwiches or wraps, or use as a topping for grilled meats or fish.

Nutrient Facts (per serving):

- Calories: 120
- Carbohydrates: 2g
- Fat: 12g
- Protein: 2g

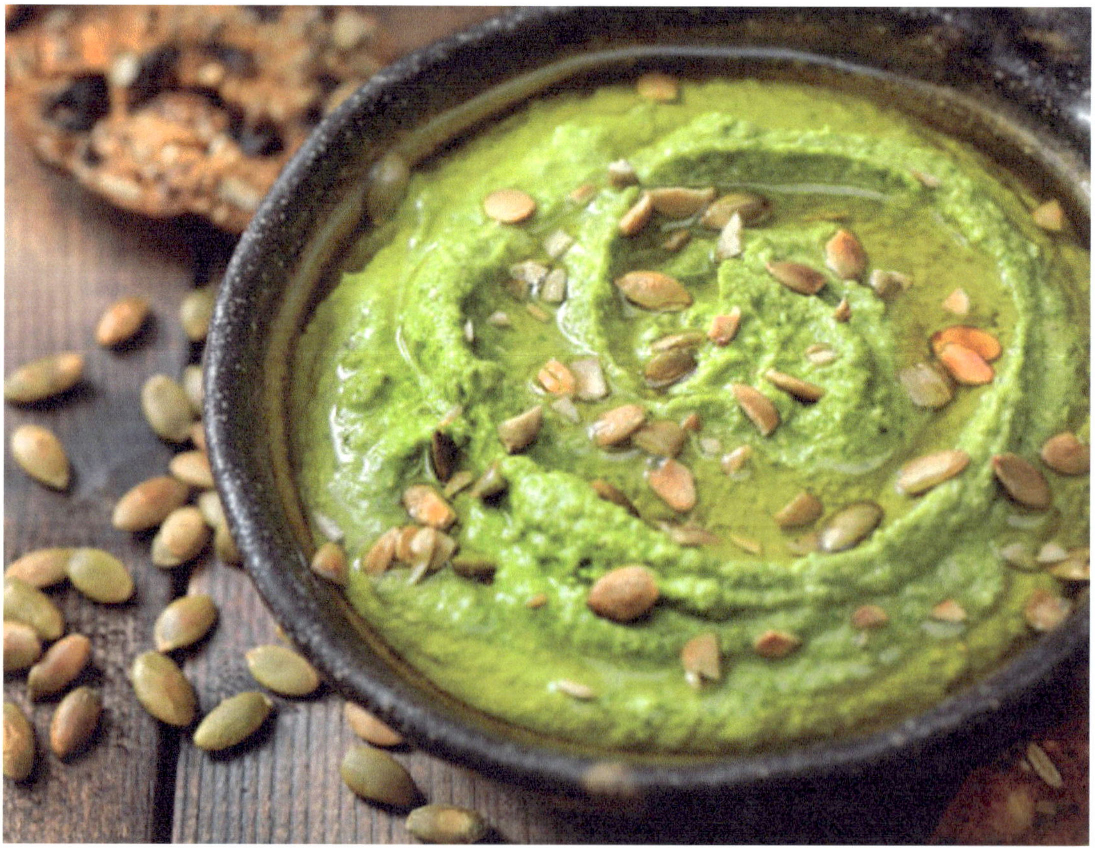

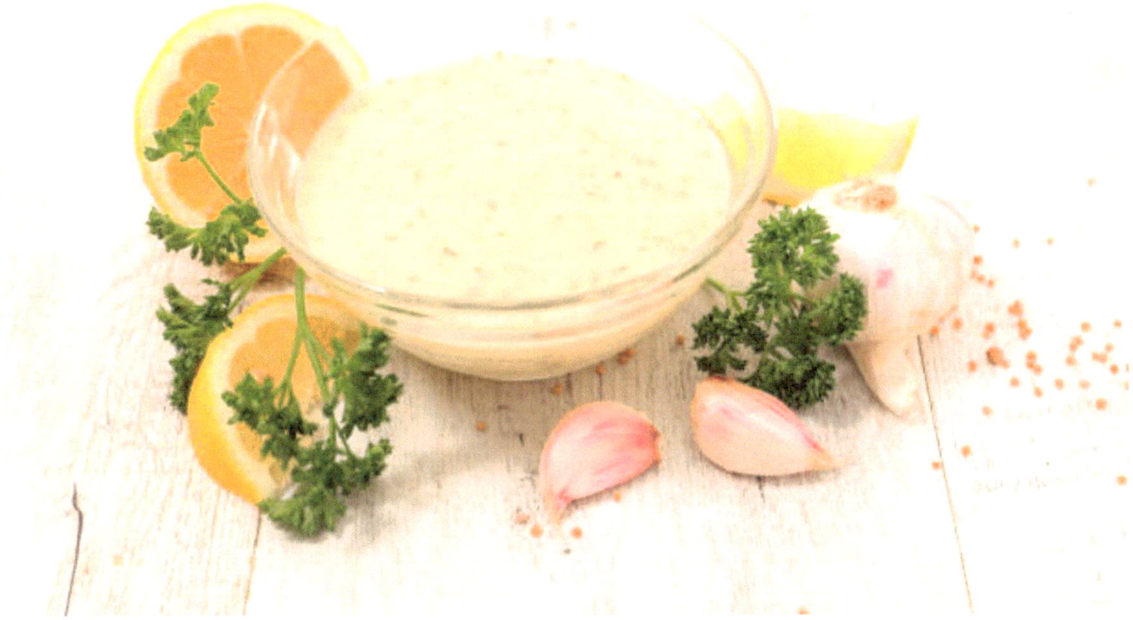

31. Lemon Garlic Yogurt Sauce

Prep.Time:	Cook Time:	Serving:
5 min	0 min	4

Ingredients:

- 1/2 cup Greek yogurt (low-fat or non-fat)
- 1 tablespoon lemon juice
- 1 clove garlic, minced
- 1 tablespoon chopped fresh parsley
- Salt and pepper to taste

Preparation:

1. In a small bowl, combine Greek yogurt, lemon juice, minced garlic, and chopped parsley.
2. Stir well to combine.
3. Season with salt and pepper according to taste.
4. Taste and adjust seasoning if necessary.
5. Serve immediately as a topping for grilled chicken, fish, or roasted vegetables.

Nutrient Facts (per serving):

- Calories: 40
- Carbohydrates: 3g
- Fat: 2g
- Protein: 3g

32. Sesame Ginger Dressing

Prep.Time: 5 min | **Cook Time:** 0 min | **Serving:** 4

Ingredients:

- 2 tablespoons sesame oil
- 2 tablespoons rice vinegar
- 1 tablespoon soy sauce (low-sodium, if preferred)
- 1 tablespoon honey or maple syrup
- 1 teaspoon grated fresh ginger
- 1 clove garlic, minced
- 1 tablespoon sesame seeds

Preparation:

1. In a small bowl, whisk together sesame oil, rice vinegar, soy sauce, honey or maple syrup, grated ginger, minced garlic, and sesame seeds until well combined.
2. Taste and adjust seasoning if necessary.
3. Serve immediately over salads, grilled vegetables, or use as a marinade for tofu or chicken.

Nutrient Facts (per serving):

- Calories: 70
- Carbohydrates: 4g
- Fat: 6g
- Protein: 1g

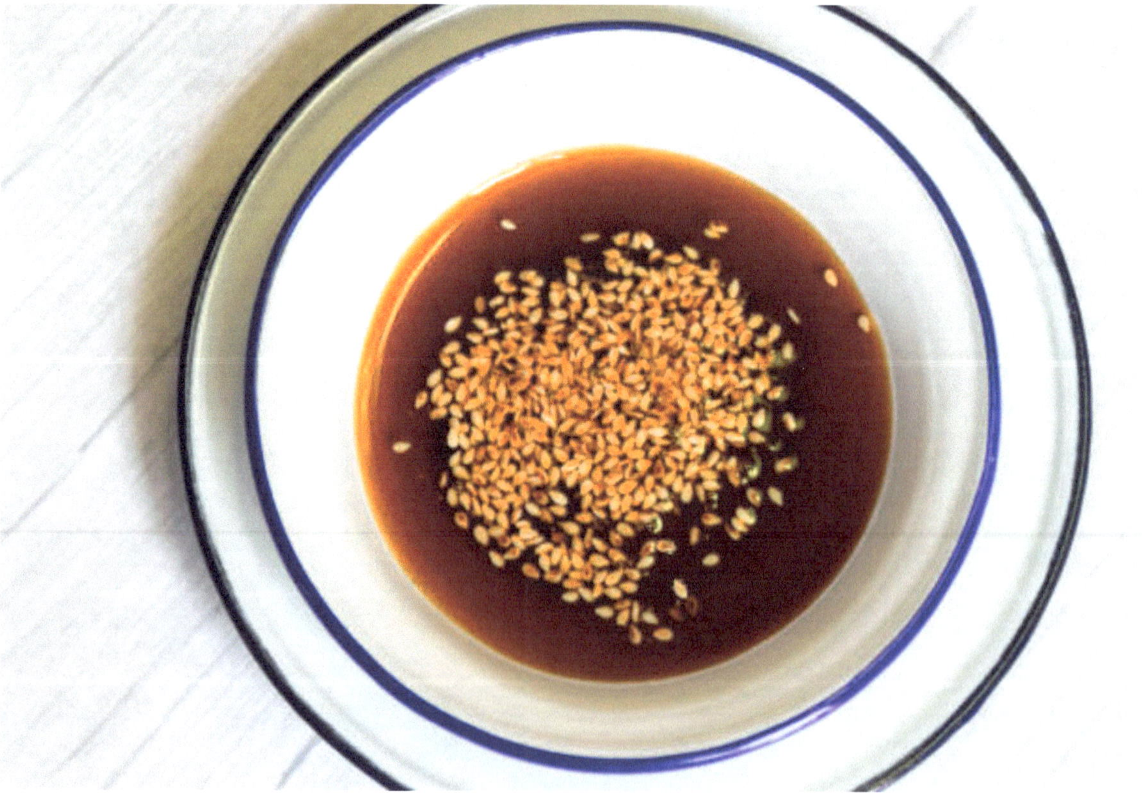

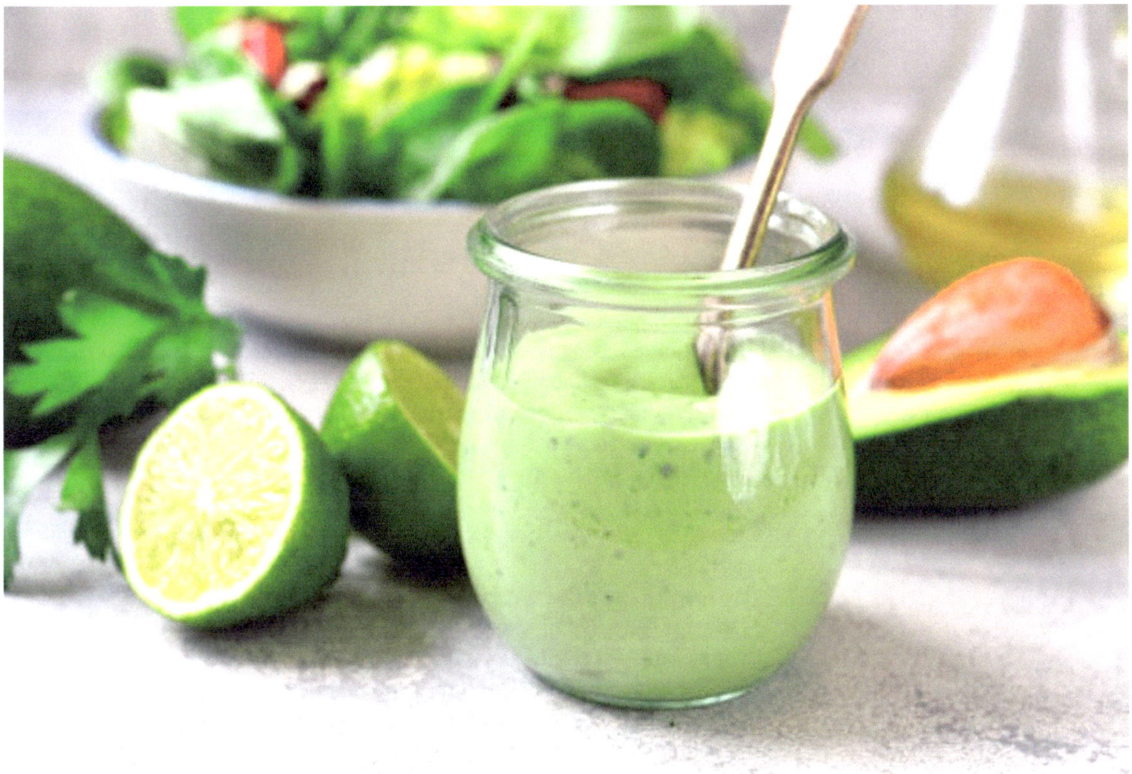

33. Creamy Avocado Cilantro Lime Dressing

Prep.Time:	Cook Time:	Serving:
10 min	0 min	4

Ingredients:

- 1 ripe avocado
- 1/4 cup Greek yogurt (low-fat or non-fat)
- 2 tablespoons chopped fresh cilantro
- 2 tablespoons lime juice
- 1 clove garlic, minced
- 1/4 teaspoon ground cumin
- Salt and pepper to taste

Preparation:

1. In a food processor or blender, combine ripe avocado, Greek yogurt, chopped cilantro, lime juice, minced garlic, and ground cumin.
2. Blend until smooth and creamy.
3. Season with salt and pepper according to taste.
4. Taste and adjust seasoning if necessary.
5. Serve immediately over salads, grilled vegetables, or as a dip for vegetable sticks or tortilla chips.

Nutrient Facts (per serving):

- Calories: 90
- Carbohydrates: 5g
- Fat: 8g
- Protein: 1g

34. Roasted Tomato Salsa

Prep.Time: 10 min

Cook Time: 25 min

Serving: 4

Ingredients:

- 3 tomatoes, halved
- 1 jalapeño pepper, halved and seeded
- 1/2 onion, peeled and quartered
- 2 cloves garlic, peeled
- 1 tablespoon olive oil
- 1 tablespoon lime juice
- 1/4 cup chopped fresh cilantro
- Salt and pepper to taste

Preparation:

1. Preheat the oven to 400°F (200°C).
2. Place halved tomatoes, halved jalapeño pepper, quartered onion, and peeled garlic cloves on a baking sheet.
3. Drizzle with olive oil and season with salt and pepper.
4. Roast in the preheated oven for 20-25 minutes, or until the vegetables are charred and softened.
5. Remove from the oven and let cool slightly.
6. In a food processor, combine roasted tomatoes, jalapeño pepper, onion, and garlic.
7. Pulse until the salsa reaches your desired consistency.
8. Transfer the salsa to a serving bowl.
9. Stir in lime juice and chopped cilantro.
10. Season with additional salt and pepper if necessary.
11. Serve chilled or at room temperature with tortilla chips or as a topping for tacos, burritos, or grilled meats.

Nutrient Facts (per serving):

- Calories: 25
- Carbohydrates: 6g
- Fat: 0g
- Protein: 1g

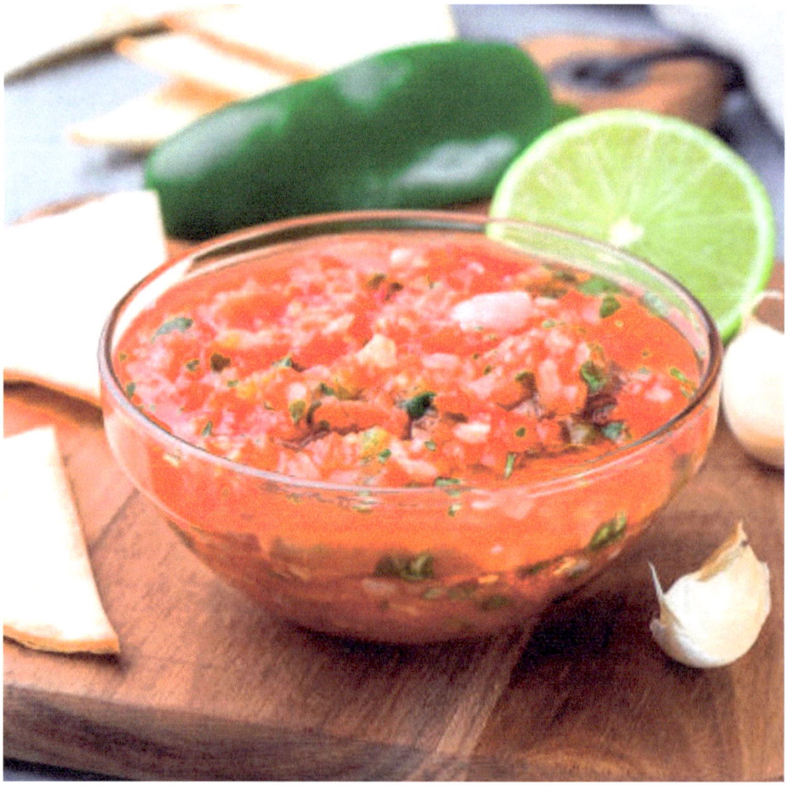

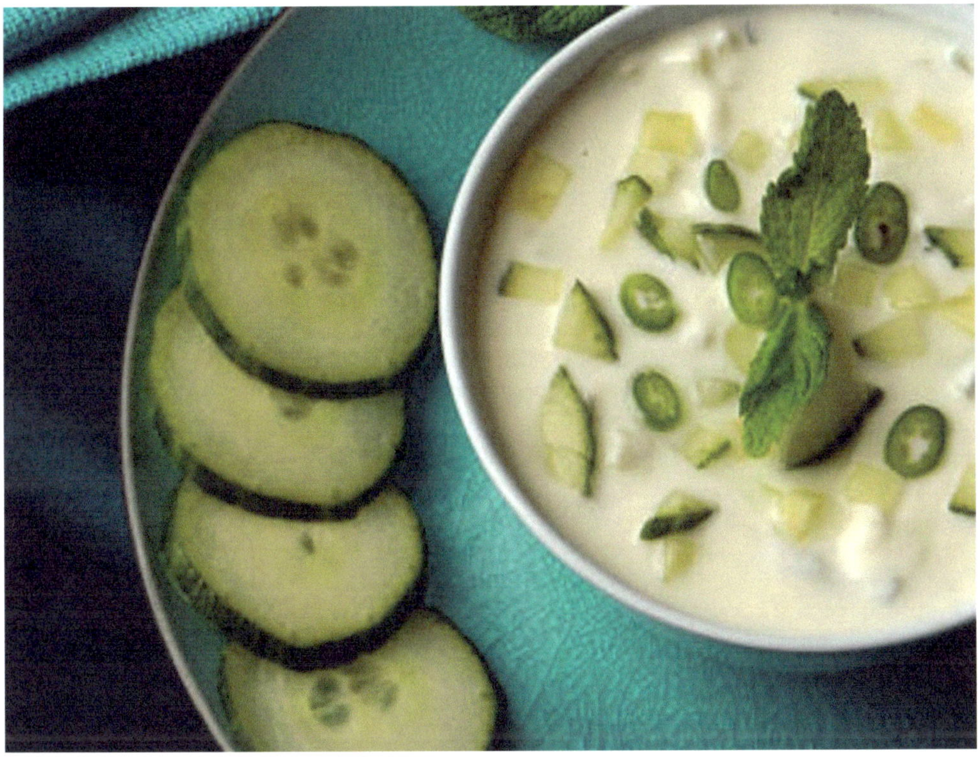

35. Cucumber Mint Yogurt Dip

Prep.Time:	Cook Time:	Serving:
10 min	0 min	4

Ingredients:

- 1/2 cup Greek yogurt (low-fat or non-fat)
- 1/2 cucumber, peeled, seeded, and finely chopped
- 1 tablespoon chopped fresh mint leaves
- 1 clove garlic, minced
- 1 tablespoon lemon juice
- Salt and pepper to taste

Preparation:

1. In a mixing bowl, combine Greek yogurt, chopped cucumber, chopped mint leaves, minced garlic, and lemon juice.
2. Stir well to combine.
3. Season with salt and pepper according to taste.
4. Taste and adjust seasoning if necessary.
5. Serve chilled with vegetable sticks, pita bread, or as a topping for grilled meats or fish.

Nutrient Facts (per serving):

- Calories: 30
- Carbohydrates: 3g
- Fat: 1g
- Protein: 2g

36. Walnut and Basil Pesto

Prep.Time: 10 min

Cook Time: 0 min

Serving: 4

Ingredients:

- 1 cup fresh basil leaves
- 1/4 cup walnuts
- 1/4 cup grated Parmesan cheese
- 1 clove garlic, minced
- 2 tablespoons lemon juice
- 1/4 cup extra virgin olive oil
- Salt and pepper to taste

Preparation:

1. In a food processor, combine basil leaves, walnuts, grated Parmesan cheese, minced garlic, and lemon juice.
2. Pulse until coarsely chopped.
3. While the food processor is running, gradually add the olive oil in a steady stream until the pesto reaches your desired consistency.
4. Season with salt and pepper according to taste.
5. Taste and adjust seasoning if necessary.
6. Transfer the pesto to a serving bowl.
7. Serve with cooked pasta, spread on sandwiches or wraps, or use as a topping for grilled meats or fish.

Nutrient Facts (per serving):

- Calories: 120
- Carbohydrates: 2g
- Fat: 12g
- Protein: 2g

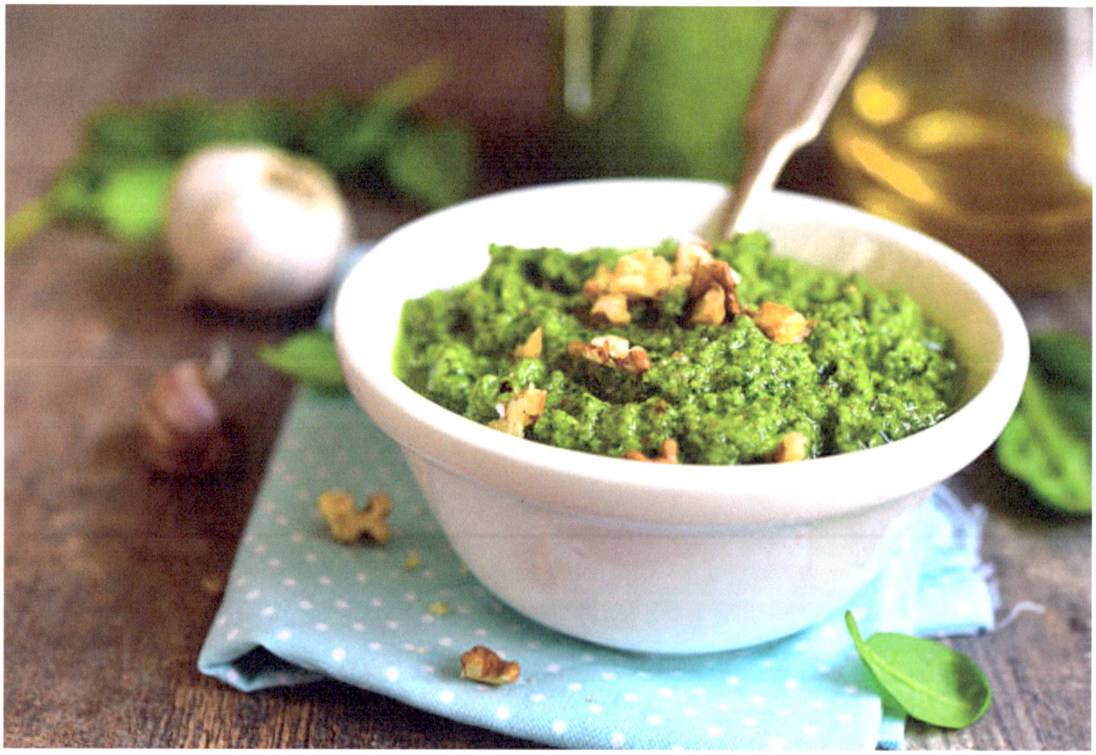

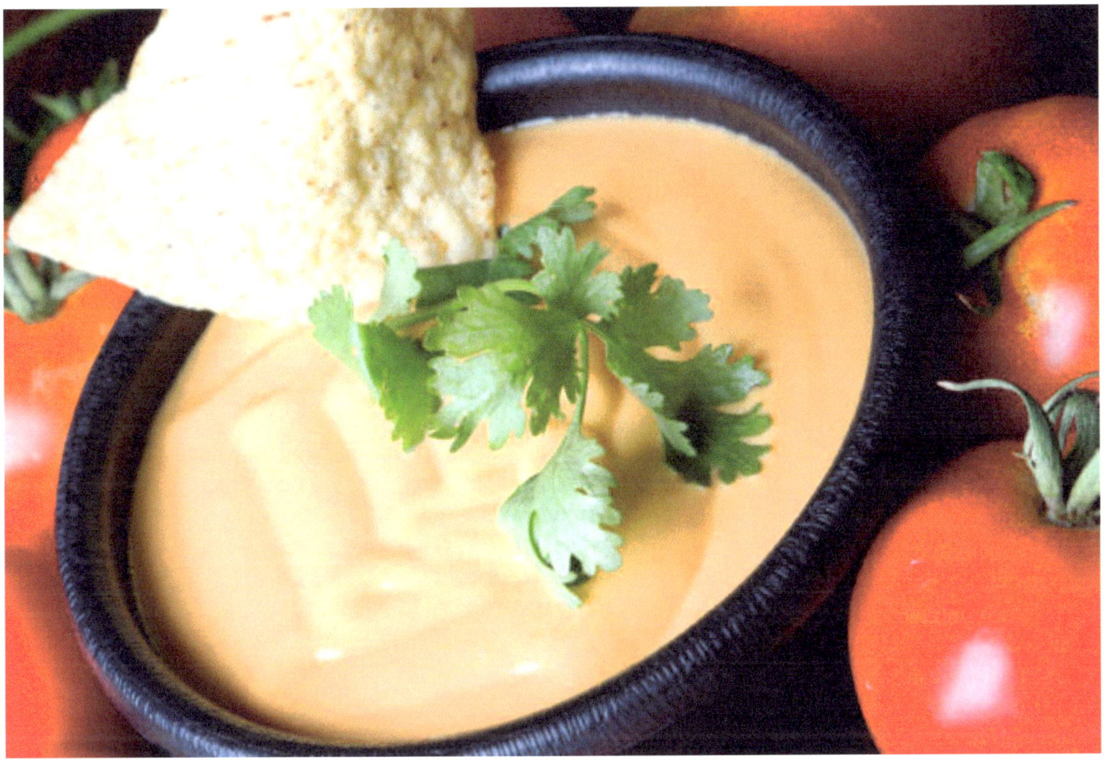

37. Spicy Chipotle Ranch Dip

Prep.Time: 5 min | **Cook Time:** 0 min | **Serving:** 4

Ingredients:

- 1/2 cup mayonnaise (light or low-fat, if preferred)
- 1/4 cup Greek yogurt (low-fat or non-fat)
- 1 chipotle pepper in adobo sauce, minced
- 1 teaspoon adobo sauce (from the chipotle peppers)
- 1 teaspoon lime juice
- 1 teaspoon chopped fresh cilantro
- 1/2 teaspoon garlic powder
- 1/2 teaspoon onion powder
- Salt and pepper to taste

Preparation:

1. In a small bowl, combine mayonnaise, Greek yogurt, minced chipotle pepper, adobo sauce, lime juice, chopped cilantro, garlic powder, and onion powder.
2. Stir well to combine.
3. Season with salt and pepper according to taste.
4. Taste and adjust seasoning if necessary.
5. Transfer to a serving bowl.
6. Serve as a dipping sauce for fries, chicken wings, or as a spread for sandwiches or wraps.

Nutrient Facts (per serving):

- Calories: 70
- Carbohydrates: 2g
- Fat: 7g
- Protein: 1g

38. Sugar-Free Ketchup

Prep.Time:	Cook Time:	Serving:
5 min	20 min	4

Ingredients:

- 1 can (6 ounces) tomato paste
- 1/4 cup apple cider vinegar
- 1 tablespoon granulated Stevia (or another sugar substitute)
- 1/2 teaspoon onion powder
- 1/2 teaspoon garlic powder
- 1/4 teaspoon salt
- 1/4 teaspoon ground black pepper
- 1/4 teaspoon ground mustard
- 1/4 teaspoon paprika
- 1/4 cup water (adjust consistency as desired)

Preparation:

1. In a saucepan, combine tomato paste, apple cider vinegar, granulated Stevia, onion powder, garlic powder, salt, black pepper, ground mustard, and paprika.
2. Stir well until smooth and fully combined.
3. Gradually add water while stirring to reach the desired consistency.
4. Bring the mixture to a simmer over medium-low heat.
5. Simmer for about 15-20 minutes, stirring occasionally, until the flavors meld and the ketchup thickens.
6. Remove from heat and let cool before serving.
7. Transfer to a glass jar or container with a lid.
8. Store in the refrigerator for up to one week

Nutrient Facts (per serving):

- Calories: 10
- Carbohydrates: 2g
- Fat: 0g
- Protein: 0g

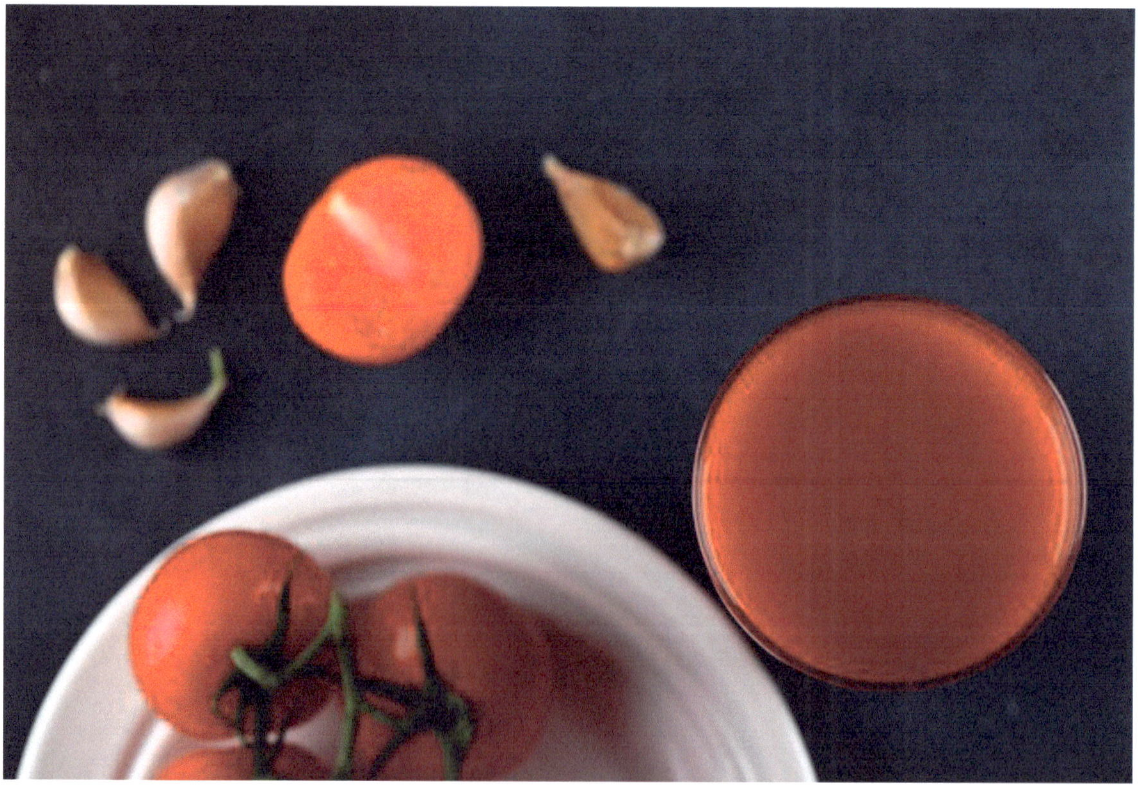

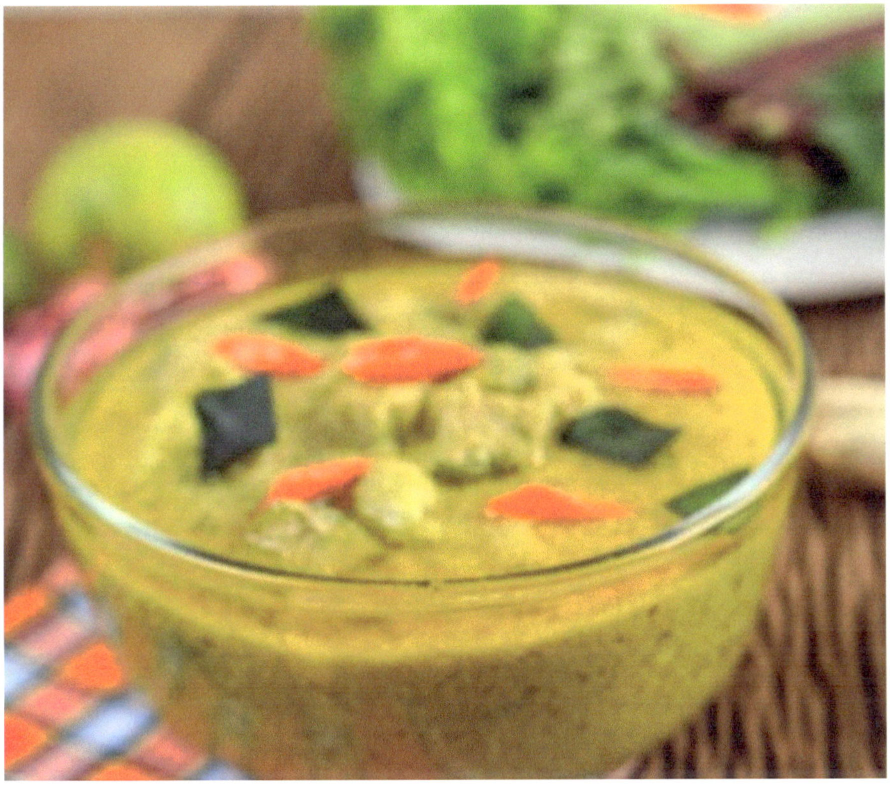

39. Mango Avocado Salsa

Prep.Time: 10 min

Cook Time: 0 min

Serving: 4

Ingredients:

- 1 ripe mango, peeled, pitted, and diced
- 1 ripe avocado, peeled, pitted, and diced
- 1/4 cup diced red onion
- 1/4 cup chopped fresh cilantro
- 1 jalapeño pepper, seeded and finely chopped
- 1 tablespoon lime juice
- Salt and pepper to taste

Preparation:

1. In a mixing bowl, combine diced mango, diced avocado, diced red onion, chopped cilantro, and chopped jalapeño pepper.
2. Drizzle with lime juice and gently toss to combine.
3. Season with salt and pepper according to taste.
4. Taste and adjust seasoning if necessary.
5. Serve immediately as a topping for grilled fish, chicken, or tacos, or with tortilla chips as a snack.

Nutrient Facts (per serving):

- Calories: 60
- Carbohydrates: 7g
- Fat: 4g
- Protein: 1g

40. Cilantro Lime Greek Yogurt Dip

Prep.Time: 5 min

Cook Time: 0 min

Serving: 4

Ingredients:

- 1/2 cup Greek yogurt (low-fat or non-fat)
- 1 tablespoon chopped fresh cilantro
- 1 tablespoon lime juice
- 1/2 teaspoon lime zest
- 1 clove garlic, minced
- Salt and pepper to taste
- Add thin slivers of carrots to taste

Preparation:

1. In a small bowl, combine Greek yogurt, chopped cilantro, lime juice, lime zest, and minced garlic.
2. Stir well to combine.
3. Season with salt and pepper according to taste.
4. Taste and adjust seasoning if necessary.
5. Serve immediately as a dip for vegetable sticks, pita chips, or as a topping for grilled meats or tacos.

Nutrient Facts (per serving):

- Calories: 40
- Carbohydrates: 3g
- Fat: 2g
- Protein: 3g

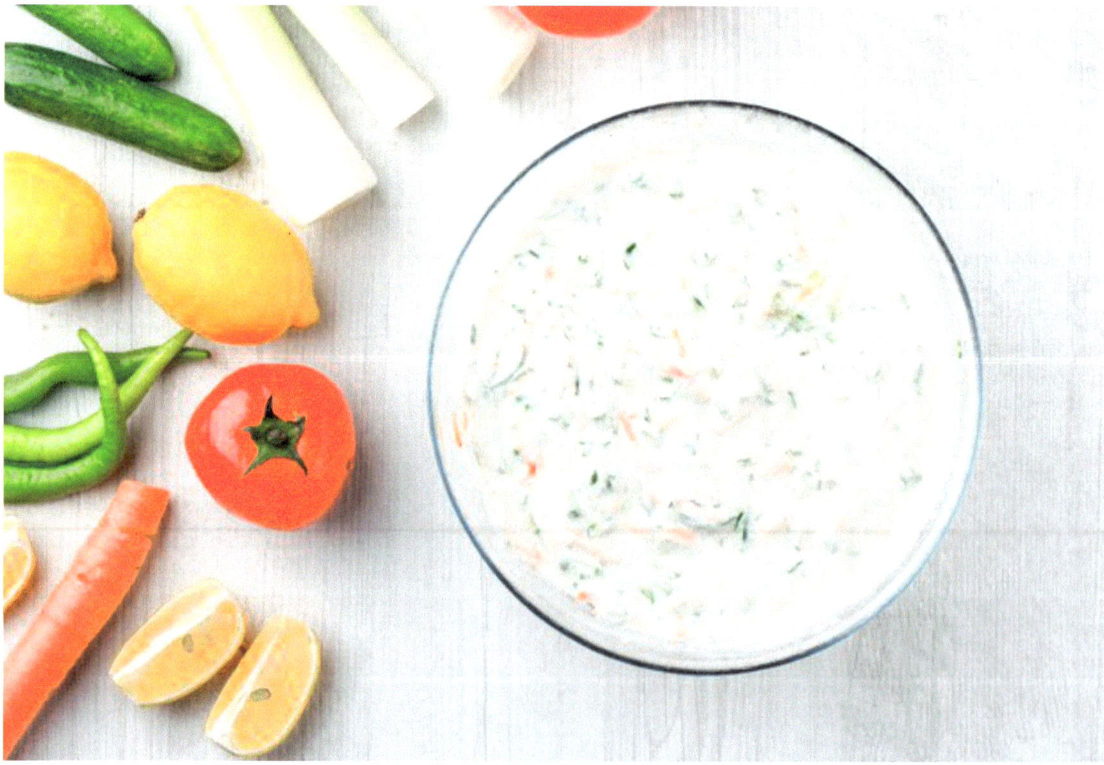

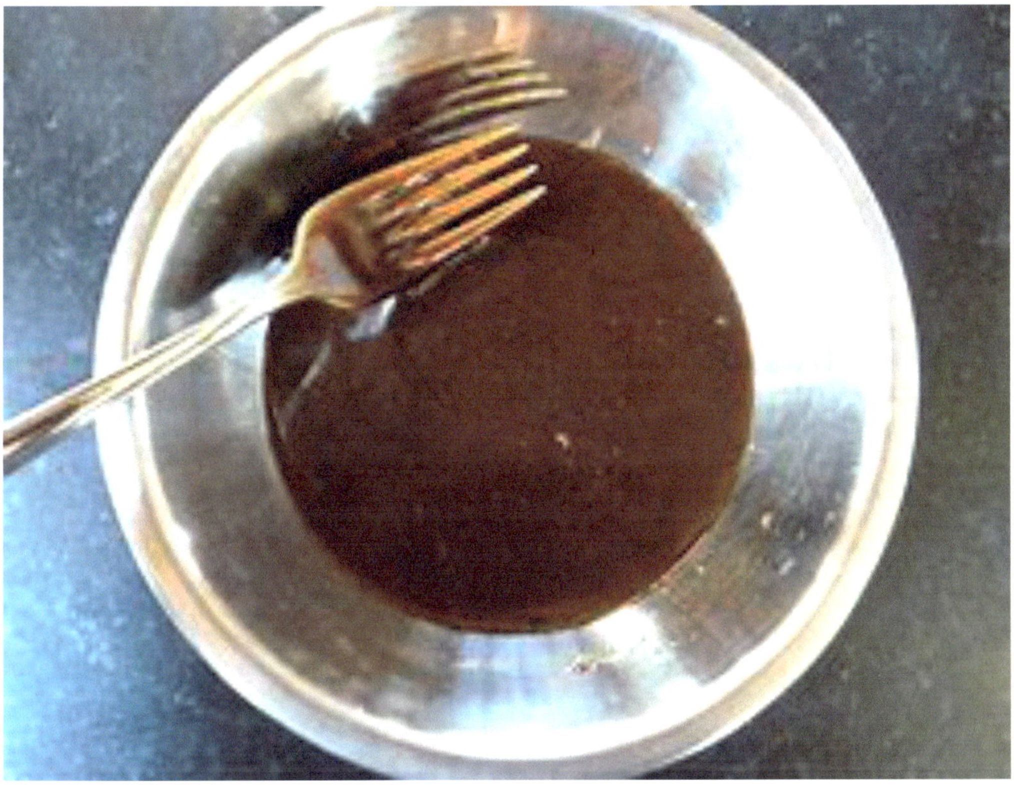

41. Balsamic Strawberry Vinaigrette

Prep.Time: 5 min | **Cook Time:** 0 min | **Serving:** 4

Ingredients:

- 1/4 cup balsamic vinegar
- 1/4 cup extra virgin olive oil
- 2 tablespoons mashed strawberries
- 1 tablespoon honey or maple syrup
- 1/2 teaspoon Dijon mustard
- Salt and pepper to taste

Preparation:

1. In a small bowl, whisk together balsamic vinegar, extra virgin olive oil, mashed strawberries, honey or maple syrup, and Dijon mustard until well combined.
2. Season with salt and pepper according to taste.
3. Taste and adjust seasoning if necessary.
4. Serve immediately over salads or grilled vegetables.

Nutrient Facts (per serving):

- Calories: 60
- Carbohydrates: 6g
- Fat: 4g
- Protein: 0g

42. Roasted Garlic and Herb Hummus

Prep.Time: 10 min | **Cook Time:** 25 min | **Serving:** 4

Ingredients:

- 1 can (15 ounces) chickpeas, drained and rinsed
- 1 head garlic
- 2 tablespoons lemon juice
- 2 tablespoons tahini (sesame seed paste)
- 1 tablespoon extra virgin olive oil
- 1 teaspoon dried parsley
- 1/2 teaspoon dried oregano
- 1/2 teaspoon dried thyme
- Salt and pepper to taste

Preparation:

1. Preheat the oven to 400°F (200°C).
2. Slice off the top of the garlic head to expose the cloves.
3. Place the garlic head on a piece of aluminum foil and drizzle with a little olive oil.
4. Wrap the garlic in the foil and place it on a baking sheet.
5. Roast in the preheated oven for 25-30 minutes, or until the garlic cloves are soft and golden brown. Remove from the oven and let cool slightly.
6. Squeeze the roasted garlic cloves out of their skins into a food processor.
7. Add drained and rinsed chickpeas, lemon juice, tahini, extra virgin olive oil, dried parsley, dried oregano, and dried thyme to the food processor.
8. Process until smooth and creamy, adding a little water if necessary to reach the desired consistency. Season with salt and pepper according to taste.
9. Taste and adjust seasoning if necessary. Transfer the hummus to a serving bowl. Serve with pita bread, vegetable sticks, or as a spread for sandwiches or wraps.

Nutrient Facts (per serving):

- Calories: 70
- Carbohydrates: 7g
- Fat: 4g
- Protein: 2g

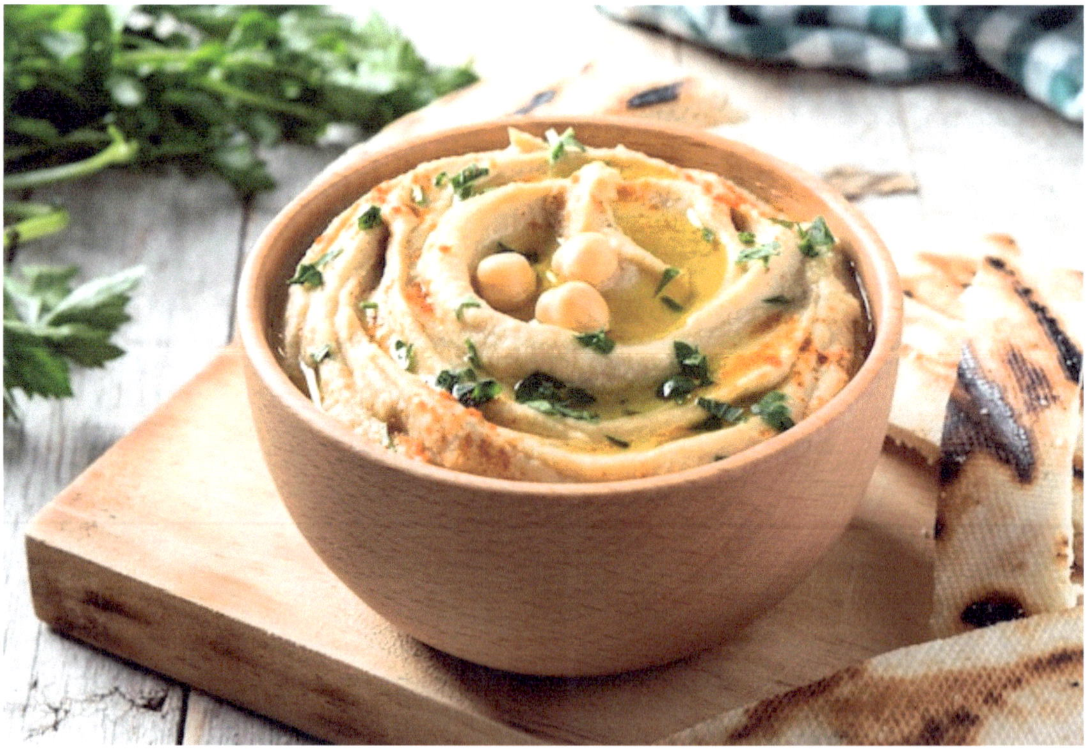

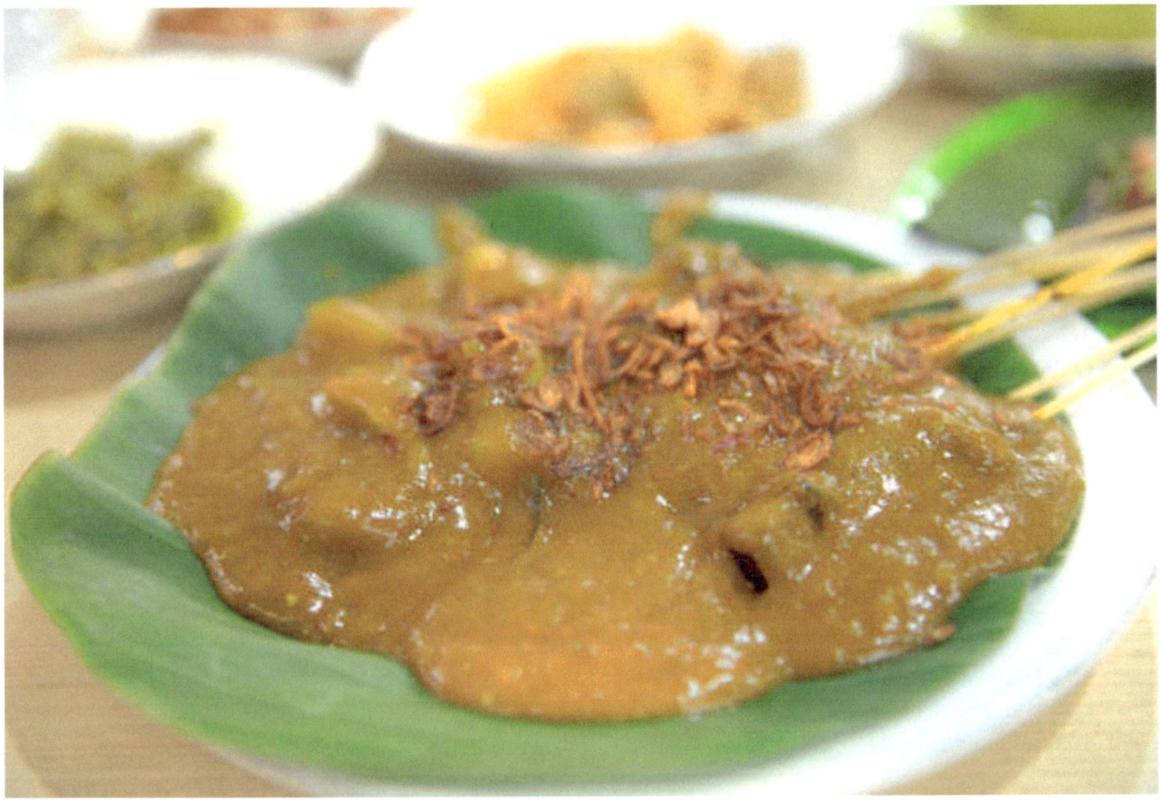

43. Peanut Sauce with Coconut Milk

Prep.Time: 10 min | **Cook Time:** 5 min | **Serving:** 4

Ingredients:

- 1/4 cup creamy peanut butter
- 1/2 cup coconut milk
- 2 tablespoons soy sauce (low-sodium, if preferred)
- 1 tablespoon lime juice
- 1 tablespoon honey or maple syrup
- 1 clove garlic, minced
- 1/2 teaspoon grated fresh ginger
- Pinch of red pepper flakes (optional)
- Salt to taste

Preparation:

1. In a small saucepan, combine creamy peanut butter, coconut milk, soy sauce, lime juice, honey or maple syrup, minced garlic, grated ginger, and red pepper flakes (if using).
2. Cook over low heat, stirring constantly, until the peanut butter is melted and the sauce is smooth.
3. Remove from heat and let cool slightly.
4. Taste and adjust seasoning with salt if necessary.
5. Serve warm or at room temperature as a dipping sauce for spring rolls, satay, or as a sauce for noodles or stir-fries.

Nutrient Facts (per serving):

- Calories: 120
- Carbohydrates: 4g
- Fat: 10g
- Protein: 3g

44. Green Goddess Dressing

Prep.Time: 10 min | **Cook Time:** 0 min | **Serving:** 4

Ingredients:

- 1/2 cup Greek yogurt (low-fat or non-fat)
- 1/4 cup chopped fresh parsley
- 2 tablespoons chopped fresh chives
- 2 tablespoons chopped fresh tarragon
- 1 tablespoon chopped fresh basil
- 1 tablespoon lemon juice
- 1 clove garlic, minced
- Salt and pepper to taste

Preparation:

1. In a blender or food processor, combine Greek yogurt, chopped parsley, chopped chives, chopped tarragon, chopped basil, lemon juice, and minced garlic.
2. Blend until smooth and creamy.
3. Season with salt and pepper according to taste.
4. Taste and adjust seasoning if necessary.
5. Serve immediately over salads, grilled vegetables, or as a dip for crudité.

Nutrient Facts (per serving):

- Calories: 80
- Carbohydrates: 2g
- Fat: 8g
- Protein: 1g

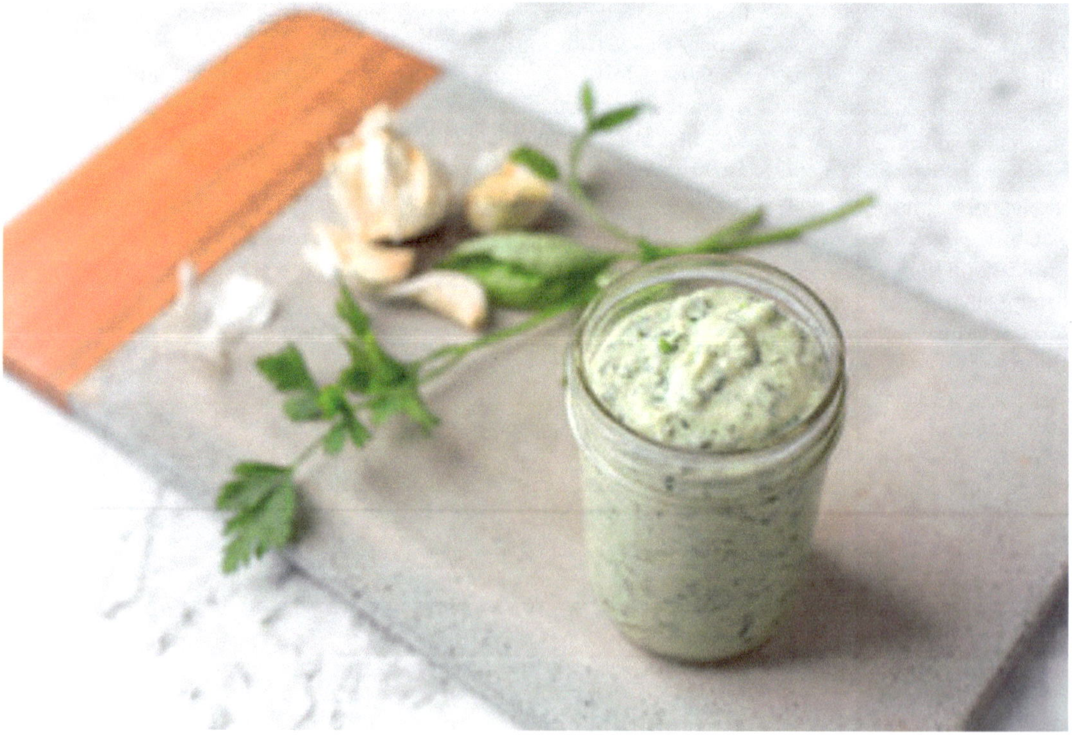

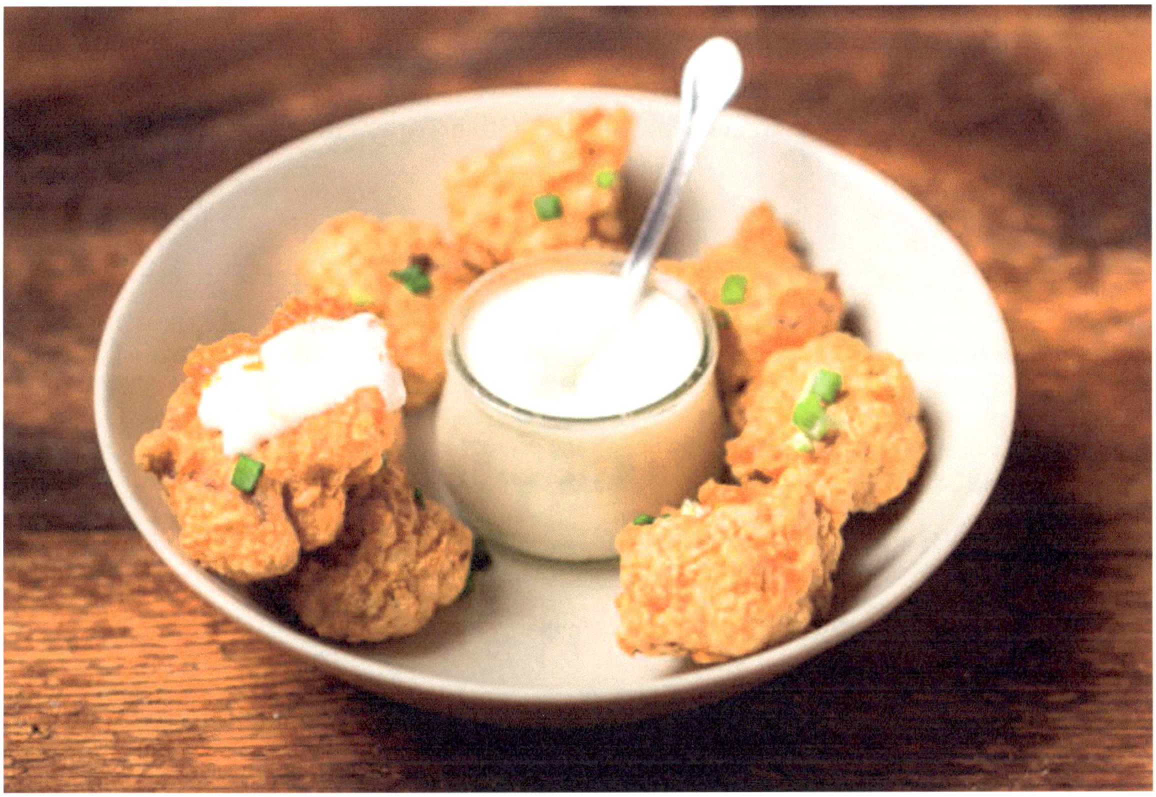

45. Cauliflower Buffalo Sauce

Prep.Time:	Cook Time:	Serving:
10 min	20 min	4

Ingredients:

- 1 cup cauliflower florets
- 1/4 cup hot sauce
- 2 tablespoons unsalted butter or vegan butter
- 1 tablespoon apple cider vinegar
- 1/2 teaspoon garlic powder
- 1/2 teaspoon onion powder
- Salt and pepper to taste

Preparation:

1. Preheat the oven to 400°F (200°C).
2. Toss cauliflower florets with a little olive oil, salt, and pepper.
3. Spread the cauliflower florets on a baking sheet and roast in the preheated oven for 15-20 minutes, or until tender and slightly browned.
4. In a small saucepan, combine hot sauce, unsalted butter or vegan butter, apple cider vinegar, garlic powder, and onion powder.
5. Cook over low heat, stirring constantly, until the butter is melted and the sauce is heated through.
6. Add the roasted cauliflower florets to the saucepan and toss to coat evenly.
7. Remove from heat and let cool slightly before serving.
8. Transfer to a serving dish.
9. Serve with celery sticks, carrot sticks, or as a topping for salads or wraps.

Nutrient Facts (per serving):

- Calories: 20
- Carbohydrates: 4g
- Fat: 0g
- Protein: 1g

46. Green Tomato and Olive Tapenade

Prep.Time: 10 min | **Cook Time:** 0 min | **Serving:** 4

Ingredients:

- 1/2 cup green tomatoes (packed in oil), drained
- 1/4 cup pitted Kalamata olives
- 2 cloves garlic, minced
- 2 tablespoons chopped fresh parsley
- 1 tablespoon lemon juice
- 2 tablespoons extra virgin olive oil
- Salt and pepper to taste

Preparation:

1. In a food processor, combine green tomatoes, pitted Kalamata olives, minced garlic, chopped parsley, lemon juice, and extra virgin olive oil.
2. Pulse until the mixture is finely chopped and reaches your desired consistency.
3. Season with salt and pepper according to taste.
4. Taste and adjust seasoning if necessary.
5. Transfer the tapenade to a serving bowl.
6. Serve with crackers, toasted bread, or as a topping for grilled fish or chicken.

Nutrient Facts (per serving):

- Calories: 80
- Carbohydrates: 4g
- Fat: 7g
- Protein: 1g

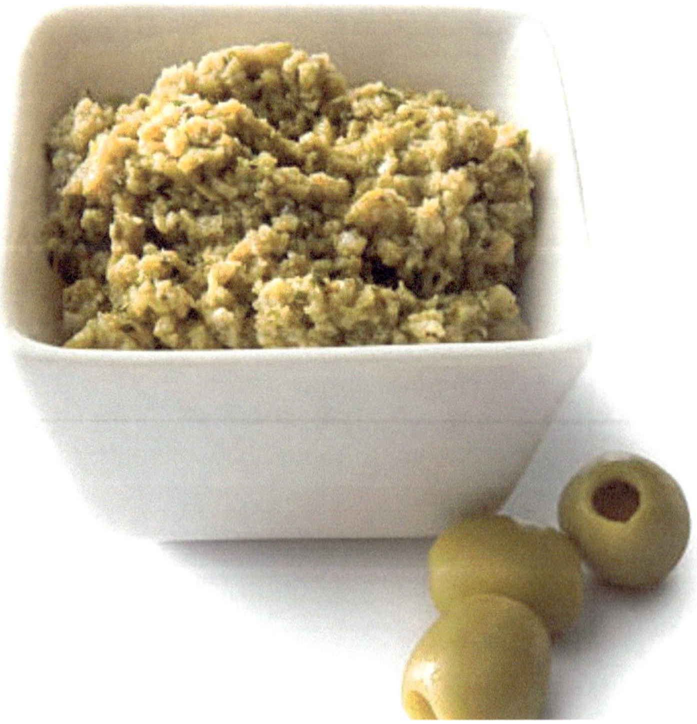

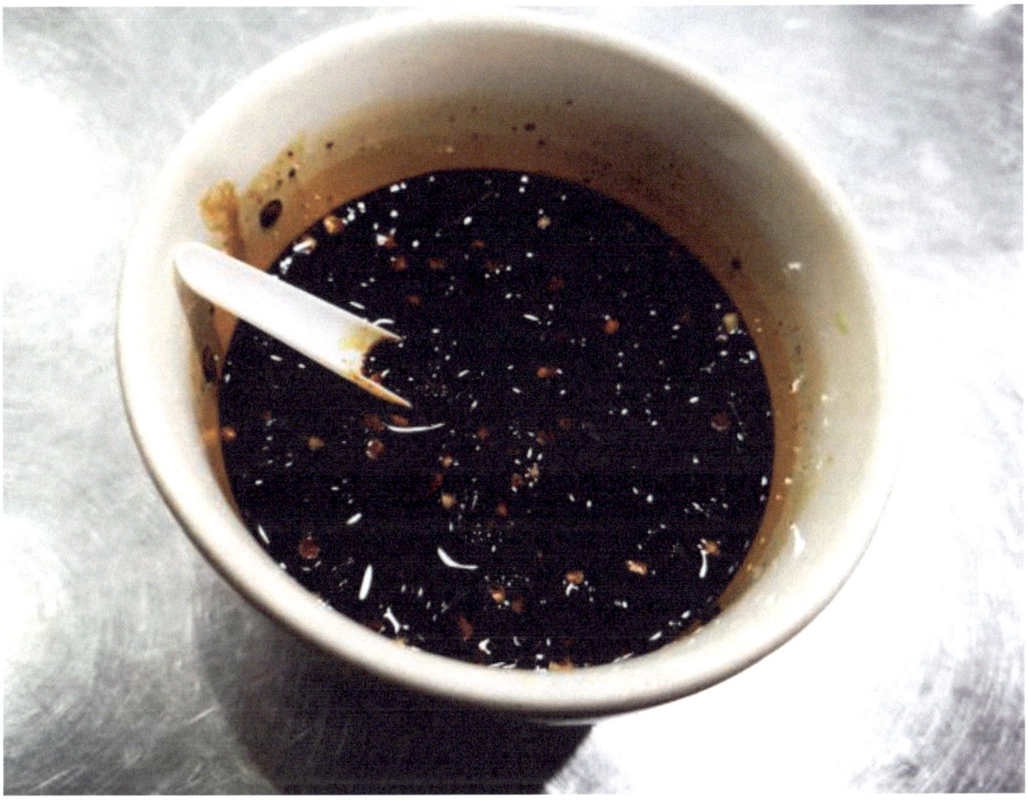

47. Soy Sesame Dipping Sauce

Prep.Time:	Cook Time:	Serving:
5 min	0 min	4

Ingredients:

- 1/4 cup soy sauce (low-sodium, if preferred)
- 2 tablespoons rice vinegar
- 1 tablespoon sesame oil
- 1 tablespoon chopped green onions
- 1 teaspoon grated fresh ginger
- 1 teaspoon honey or maple syrup
- 1/2 teaspoon sesame seeds (optional)

Preparation:

1. In a small bowl, whisk together soy sauce, rice vinegar, sesame oil, chopped green onions, grated fresh ginger, and honey or maple syrup until well combined.
2. If desired, sprinkle sesame seeds on top.
3. Serve immediately as a dipping sauce for dumplings, spring rolls, or as a marinade for grilled meats or tofu.

Nutrient Facts (per serving):

- Calories: 40
- Carbohydrates: 3g
- Fat: 2g
- Protein: 2g

48. Avocado Cilantro Lime Salsa

Prep.Time: 10 min | **Cook Time:** 0 min | **Serving:** 4

Ingredients:

- 1 ripe avocado, diced
- 1/4 cup diced red onion
- 1/4 cup chopped fresh cilantro
- 1 jalapeño pepper, seeded and finely chopped
- 1 tablespoon lime juice
- Salt and pepper to taste

Preparation:

1. In a mixing bowl, combine diced avocado, diced red onion, chopped cilantro, and chopped jalapeño pepper.
2. Drizzle with lime juice and gently toss to combine.
3. Season with salt and pepper according to taste.
4. Taste and adjust seasoning if necessary.
5. Serve immediately as a topping for grilled fish, chicken, or tacos, or with tortilla chips as a snack.

Nutrient Facts (per serving):

- Calories: 70
- Carbohydrates: 5g
- Fat: 6g
- Protein: 1g

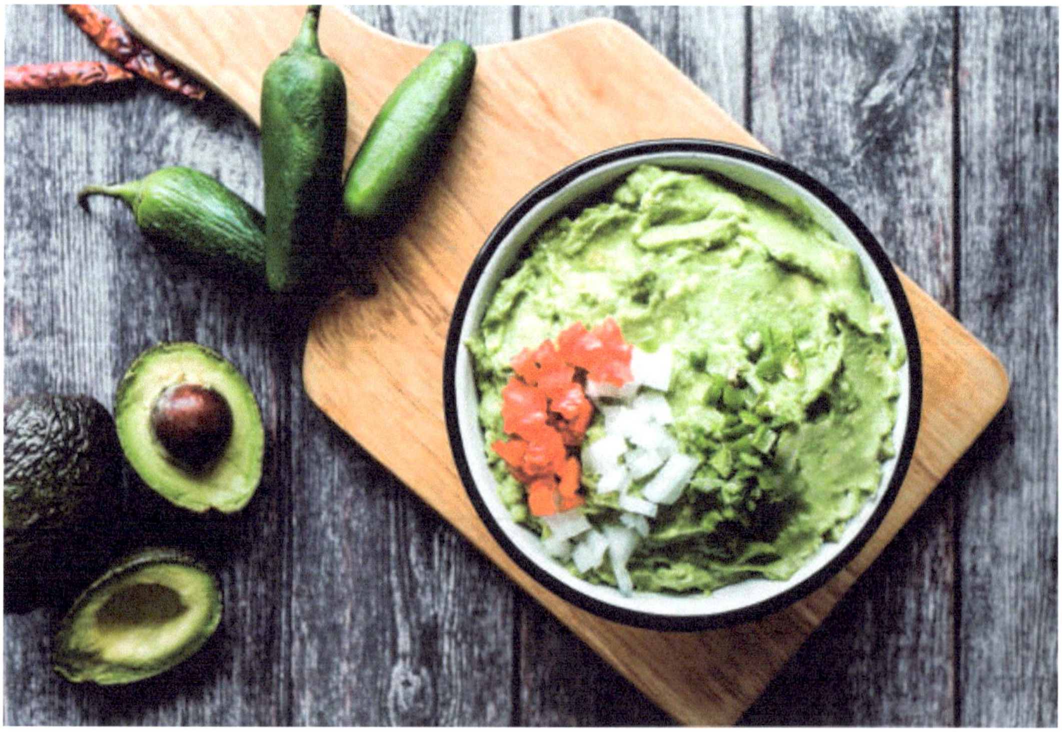

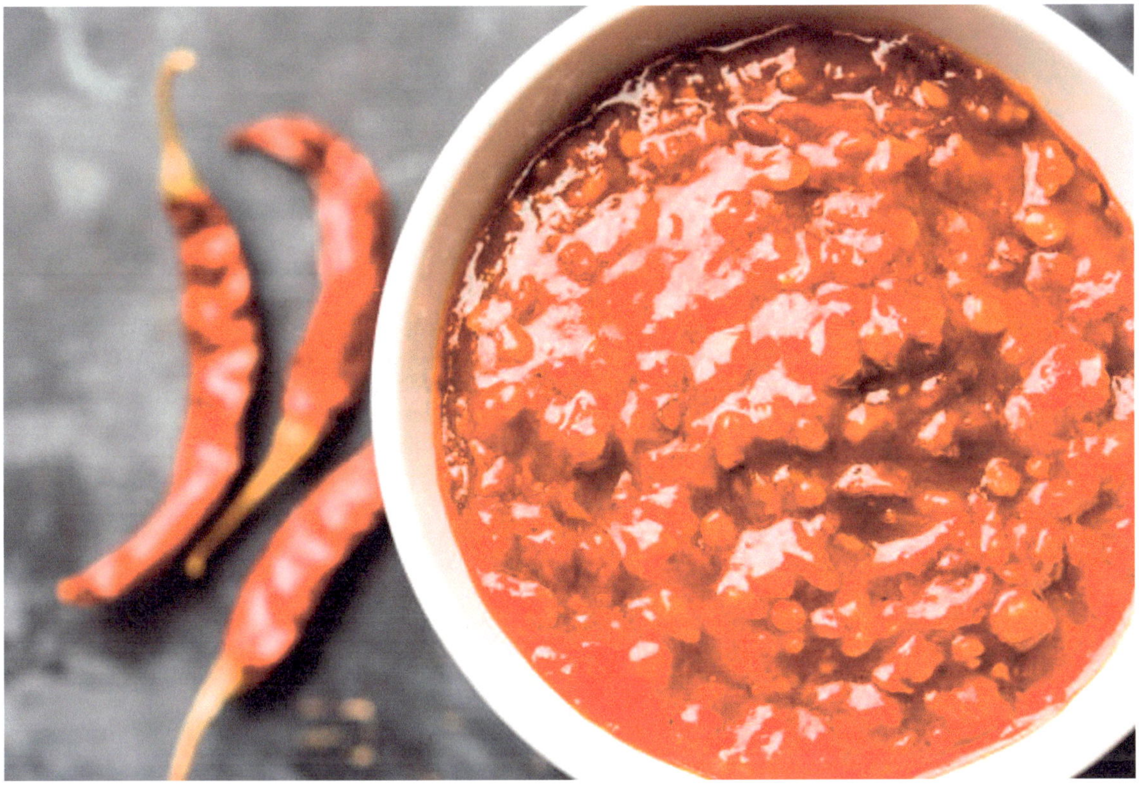

49. Low-Sugar Sweet Chili Sauce

Prep.Time: 5 min | **Cook Time:** 10 min | **Serving:** 4

Ingredients:

- 1/2 cup water
- 1/4 cup rice vinegar
- 2 tablespoons soy sauce (low-sodium, if preferred)
- 2 tablespoons erythritol (or another sugar substitute)
- 1 tablespoon tomato paste
- 1 teaspoon minced garlic
- 1 teaspoon minced ginger
- 1 teaspoon chili flakes (adjust to taste)
- 1 teaspoon cornstarch mixed with 1 tablespoon water (optional, for thickening)

Preparation:

1. In a small saucepan, combine water, rice vinegar, soy sauce, erythritol, tomato paste, minced garlic, minced ginger, and chili flakes.
2. Stir well and bring to a simmer over medium heat.
3. Let the mixture simmer for about 5-7 minutes, stirring occasionally, until slightly thickened.
4. If desired, add the cornstarch mixture to the sauce to thicken further, stirring continuously for another 2-3 minutes.
5. Remove from heat and let cool before serving.
6. Transfer to a glass jar or container with a lid.
7. Store in the refrigerator for up to one week.

Nutrient Facts (per serving):

- Calories: 40
- Carbohydrates: 9g
- Fat: 0g
- Protein: 0g

50. Tahini Yogurt Sauce

Prep.Time: 5 min | **Cook Time:** 0 min | **Serving:** 4

Ingredients:

- 1/4 cup Greek yogurt (low-fat or non-fat)
- 2 tablespoons tahini (sesame seed paste)
- 1 tablespoon lemon juice
- 1 clove garlic, minced
- 1 tablespoon chopped fresh parsley (optional)
- Salt and pepper to taste

Preparation:

1. In a small bowl, whisk together Greek yogurt, tahini, lemon juice, minced garlic, and chopped fresh parsley (if using) until smooth and creamy.
2. Season with salt and pepper according to taste.
3. Taste and adjust seasoning if necessary.
4. Serve immediately as a sauce for falafel, grilled vegetables, or as a dip for pita bread or vegetable sticks.

Nutrient Facts (per serving):

- Calories: 60
- Carbohydrates: 3g
- Fat: 4g
- Protein: 3g

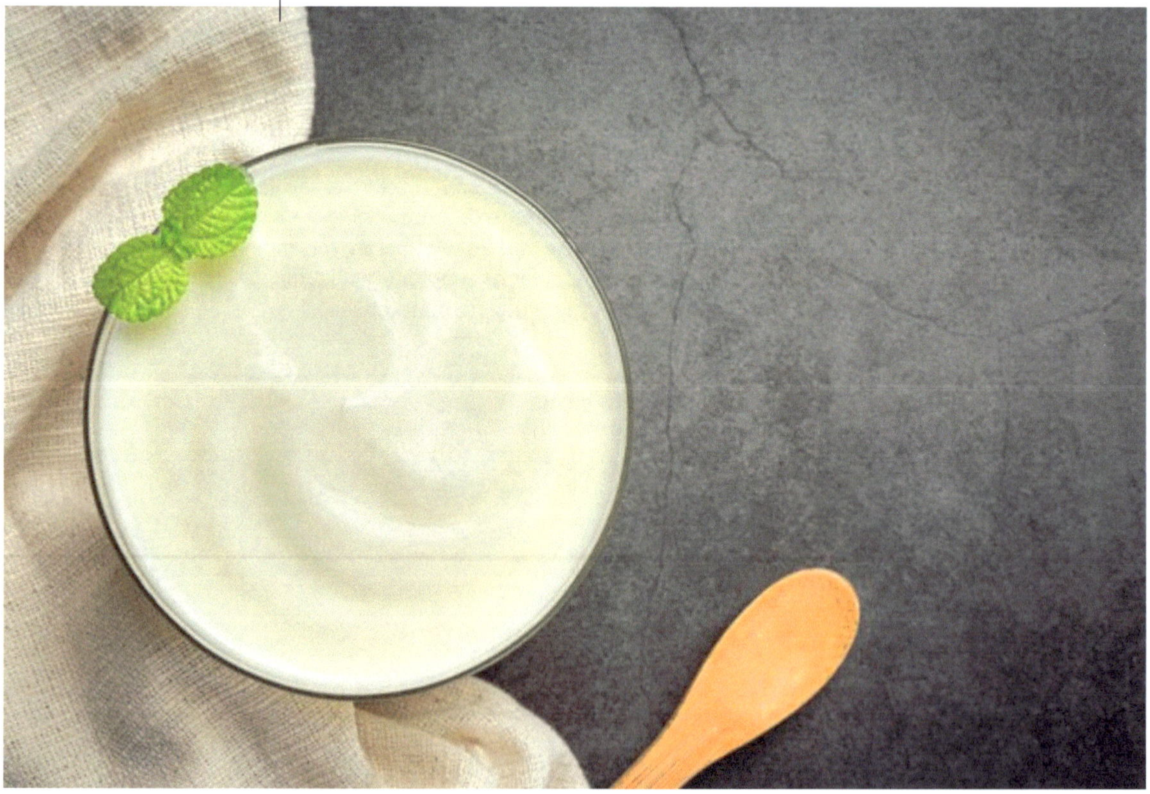

Your Kindness is Key

Share Your Experience, Share Your Strength

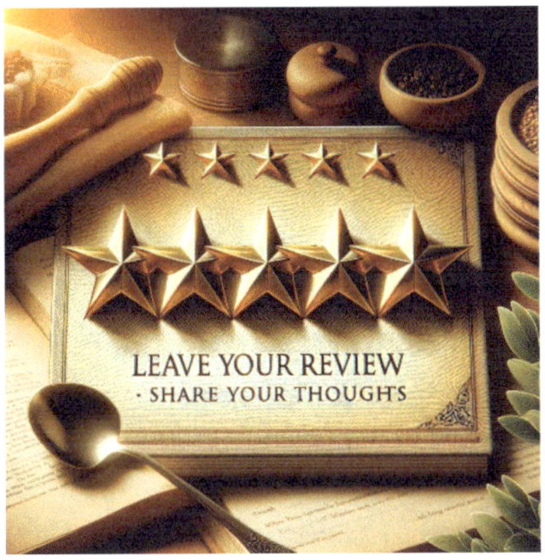

"Helping one person might not change the whole world, but it could change the world for one person." - Anonymous

---

Do you remember what it was like when you first heard the words "Type 2 Diabetes?" Perhaps it felt like a mountain you weren't sure you could climb.

Maybe it was daunting, thinking about the changes you'd have to make in your life, especially with your diet. It's a journey many embark on feeling uncertain and alone.

But you've found a companion on this journey, haven't you? Type 2 Diabetes Cookbook Beginner's Quick & Easy Recipes for Delicious Diabetes Diets by Lily Anders has been with you, offering guidance, delicious recipes, and a sense of control over your diabetes that perhaps you didn't feel before.

Imagine if you could light the path for someone just starting on this journey. Someone who feels lost in the sea of information, unsure of where to turn for reliable, practical advice on managing their diabetes through diet. Your experience, shared through a review, could be the beacon they need.

This isn't just about leaving a review; it's about extending a hand, offering support, and sharing the strength that comes from knowledge and community. Your words could help another person find their footing, making their journey a bit easier and less lonely.

So, here's my humble request on behalf of a fellow journeyer you've yet to meet:

Please take a moment to share your experience with the book. Your insights could be the very thing another person needs to hear to take that first, brave step toward a healthier, happier life with diabetes. Your review, a simple act of kindness, asks for nothing in return yet offers immeasurable value.

To leave your review, just follow this link:

https://www.amazon.com/review/create-review/?ie=UTF8&channel=glance-detail&asin=1963939344

If the thought of helping another soul on their diabetes journey warms your heart, then you're exactly who I hoped to reach with this book. Welcome to a community where kindness, support, and shared victories pave the way to a better life.

I'm beyond grateful for your help in spreading the word and even more excited to continue providing you with the knowledge and recipes to make managing diabetes not just manageable, but enjoyable.

Click the QR Code Here!

Thank you from the deepest places in my heart. Your generosity makes all the difference.

Lily Anders

P.S. - Sharing is caring, they say. If you believe this book has brought value to your life and could do the same for someone else, consider sharing it with them. It's another beautiful way to change a life, one meal at a time.

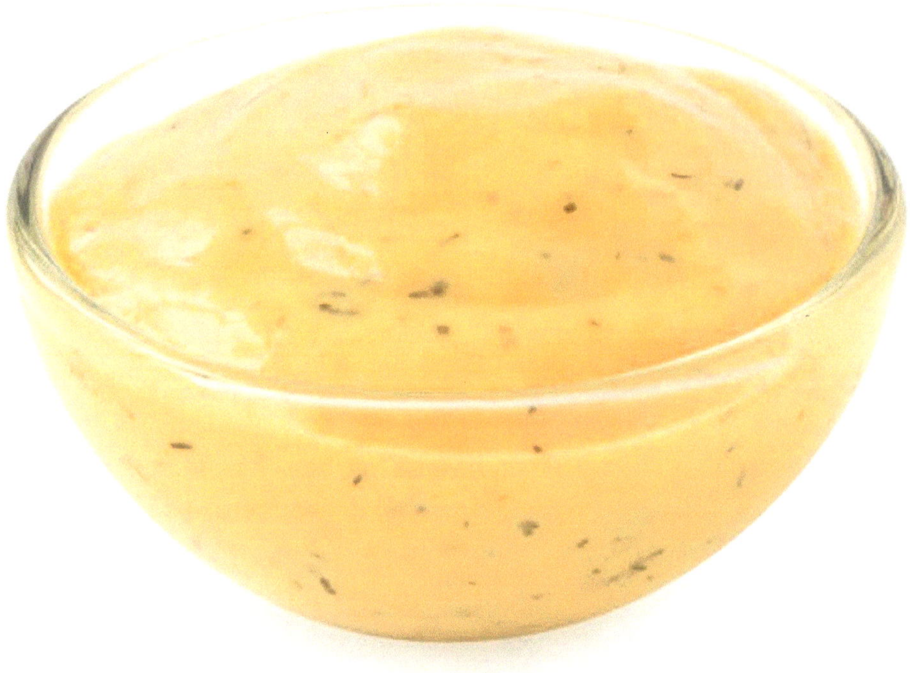

51. Sugar-Free Dijon Mustard Dressing

Prep.Time:	Cook Time:	Serving:
5 min	0 min	4

Ingredients:

- 2 tablespoons Dijon mustard
- 2 tablespoons apple cider vinegar
- 2 tablespoons extra virgin olive oil
- 1 teaspoon erythritol (or another sugar substitute)
- 1 clove garlic, minced
- Salt and pepper to taste

Preparation:

1. In a small bowl, whisk together Dijon mustard, apple cider vinegar, extra virgin olive oil, erythritol, minced garlic, salt, and pepper until well combined.
2. Taste and adjust seasoning if necessary.
3. Serve immediately over salads, roasted vegetables, or grilled meats

Nutrient Facts (per serving):

- Calories: 30
- Carbohydrates: 1g
- Fat: 3g
- Protein: 0g

52. Cucumber and Radish Yogurt Dip

Prep.Time: 10 min

Cook Time: 0 min

Serving: 4

Ingredients:

- 1/2 cup Greek yogurt (low-fat or non-fat)
- 1/2 cup diced cucumber
- 1/4 cup diced radishes
- 1 tablespoon chopped fresh dill
- 1 teaspoon lemon juice
- Salt and pepper to taste

Preparation:

1. In a mixing bowl, combine Greek yogurt, diced cucumber, diced radishes, chopped fresh dill, and lemon juice.
2. Stir well to combine.
3. Season with salt and pepper according to taste.
4. Taste and adjust seasoning if necessary.
5. Serve chilled with vegetable sticks, pita bread, or as a topping for grilled meats or fish.

Nutrient Facts (per serving):

- Calories: 30
- Carbohydrates: 3g
- Fat: 1g
- Protein: 2g

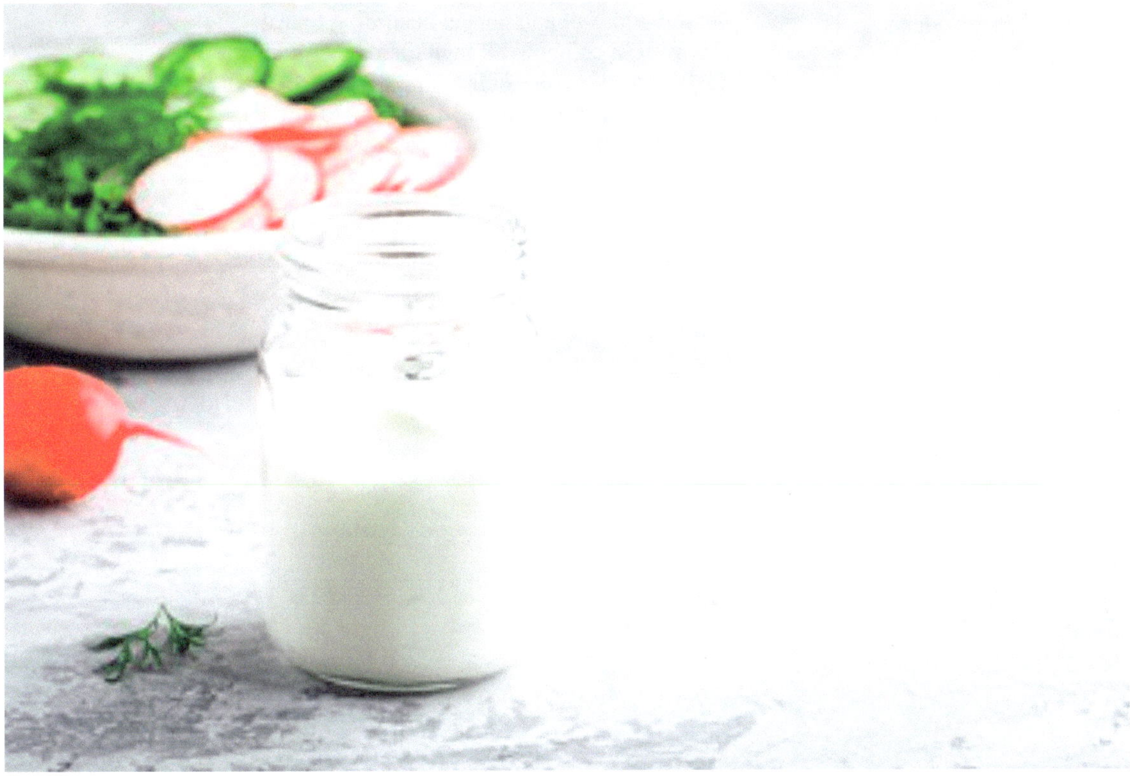

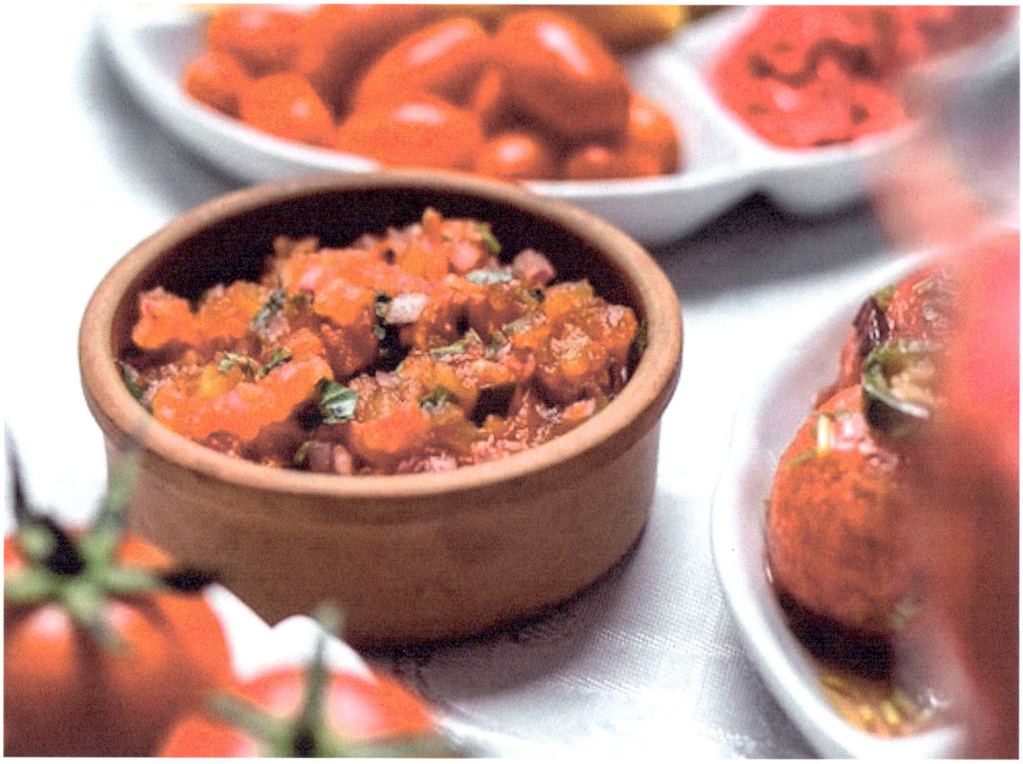

53. Smoky Chipotle Tomato Salsa

Prep.Time: 10 min | **Cook Time:** 10 min | **Serving:** 4

Ingredients:

- 2 large tomatoes, diced
- 1 chipotle pepper in adobo sauce, minced
- 1/4 cup diced red onion
- 2 tablespoons chopped fresh cilantro
- 1 tablespoon lime juice
- 1/2 teaspoon smoked paprika
- Salt and pepper to taste

Preparation:

1. In a bowl, combine diced tomatoes, minced chipotle pepper, diced red onion, chopped cilantro, lime juice, and smoked paprika.
2. Season with salt and pepper according to taste.
3. Mix well to combine all ingredients thoroughly.
4. Taste and adjust seasoning if necessary.
5. Let the salsa sit for about 10 minutes to allow the flavors to meld.
6. Serve chilled with tortilla chips or as a topping for tacos, burritos, or grilled meats.

Nutrient Facts (per serving):

- Calories: 25
- Carbohydrates: 6g
- Fat: 0g
- Protein: 1g

54. Lemon Herb Greek Yogurt Dressing

Prep.Time: 5 min | **Cook Time:** 0 min | **Serving:** 4

Ingredients:

- 1/2 cup Greek yogurt (low-fat or non-fat)
- 2 tablespoons lemon juice
- 1 tablespoon chopped fresh parsley
- 1 tablespoon chopped fresh dill
- 1 teaspoon minced garlic
- Salt and pepper to taste

Preparation:

1. In a mixing bowl, whisk together Greek yogurt, lemon juice, chopped parsley, chopped dill, minced garlic, salt, and pepper until smooth.
2. Taste and adjust seasoning if necessary.
3. Serve immediately over salads, grilled vegetables, or as a dip for vegetable sticks.

Nutrient Facts (per serving):

- Calories: 40
- Carbohydrates: 3g
- Fat: 2g
- Protein: 3g

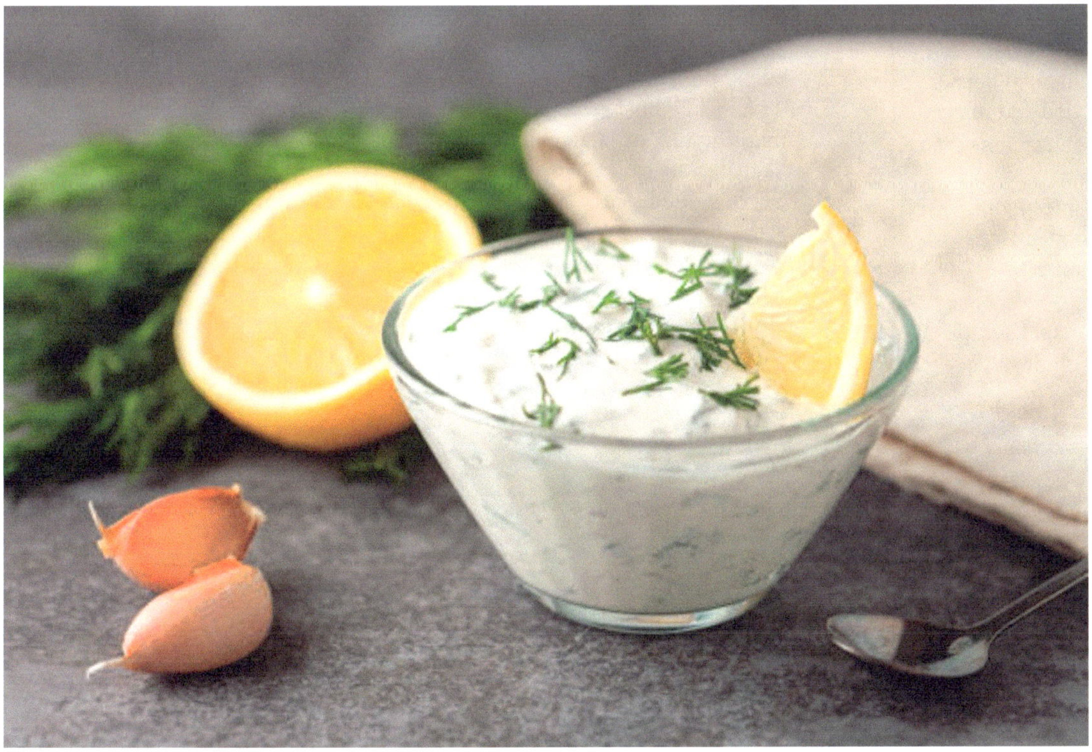

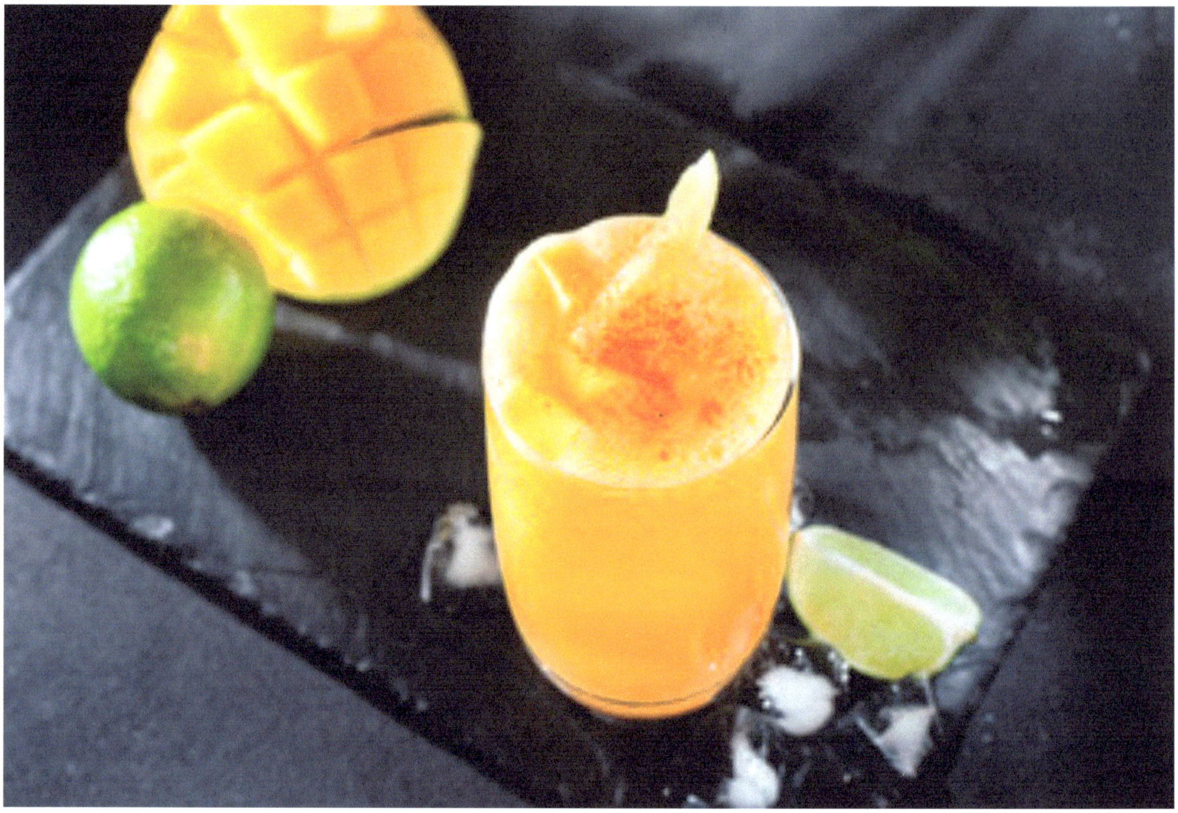

55. Mango Jalapeño Lime Sauce

Prep.Time: 10 min | **Cook Time:** 0 min | **Serving:** 4

Ingredients:

- 1 ripe mango, peeled, pitted, and diced
- 1 jalapeño pepper, seeded and minced
- 2 tablespoons lime juice
- 1 tablespoon chopped fresh cilantro
- 1 teaspoon honey or maple syrup
- Pinch of salt

Preparation:

1. In a blender or food processor, combine diced mango, minced jalapeño pepper, lime juice, chopped cilantro, honey or maple syrup, and a pinch of salt.
2. Blend until smooth.
3. Taste and adjust sweetness or spiciness if desired by adding more honey, maple syrup, or jalapeño pepper.
4. Transfer the sauce to a serving bowl.
5. Serve chilled as a topping for grilled fish, chicken, or tacos, or as a dipping sauce for spring rolls or shrimp.

Nutrient Facts (per serving):

- Calories: 50
- Carbohydrates: 12g
- Fat: 0g
- Protein: 1g

56. Cilantro Lime Coconut Aminos Dressing

Prep.Time: 5 min

Cook Time: 0 min

Serving: 4

Ingredients:

- 2 tablespoons coconut aminos
- 2 tablespoons lime juice
- 2 tablespoons chopped fresh cilantro
- 1 tablespoon extra virgin olive oil
- 1 teaspoon minced garlic
- 1 teaspoon honey or maple syrup
- Salt and pepper to taste

Preparation:

1. In a small bowl, whisk together coconut aminos, lime juice, chopped cilantro, extra virgin olive oil, minced garlic, honey or maple syrup, salt, and pepper until well combined.
2. Taste and adjust seasoning if necessary.
3. Serve immediately over salads, rice bowls, or grilled vegetables.

Nutrient Facts (per serving):

- Calories: 60
- Carbohydrates: 5g
- Fat: 4g
- Protein: 1g

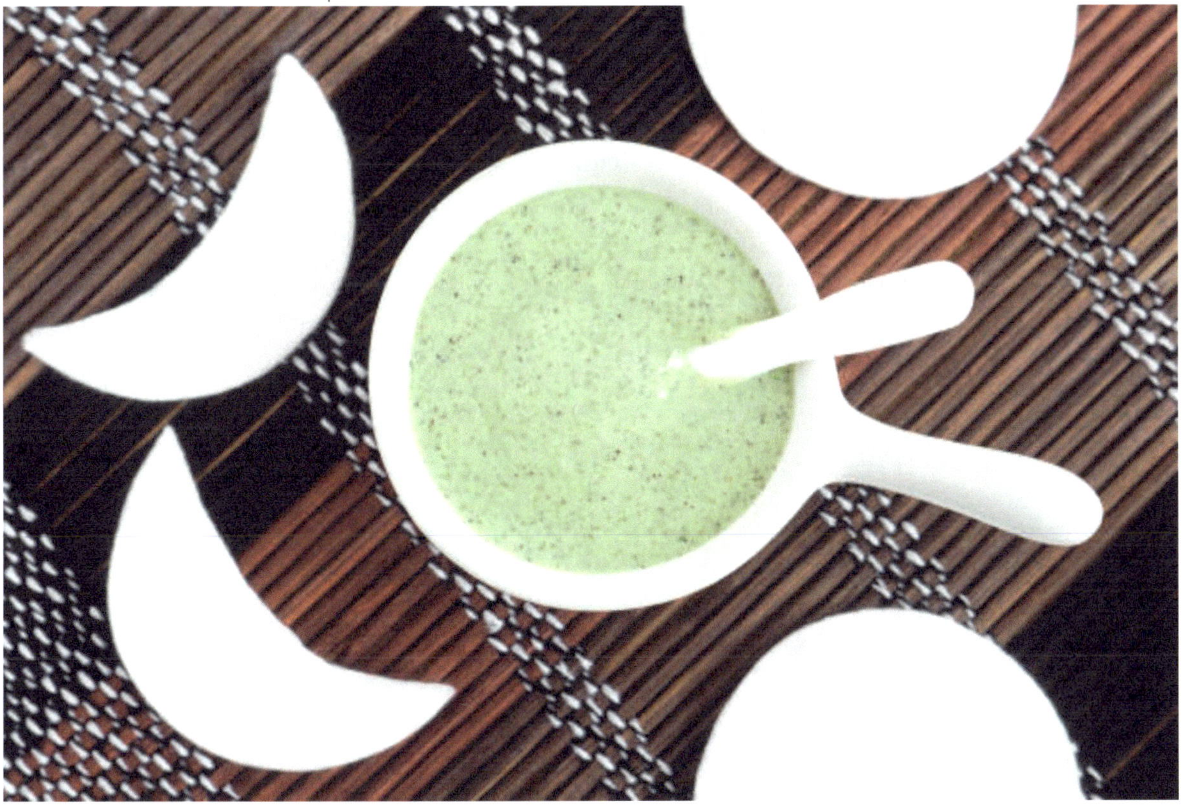

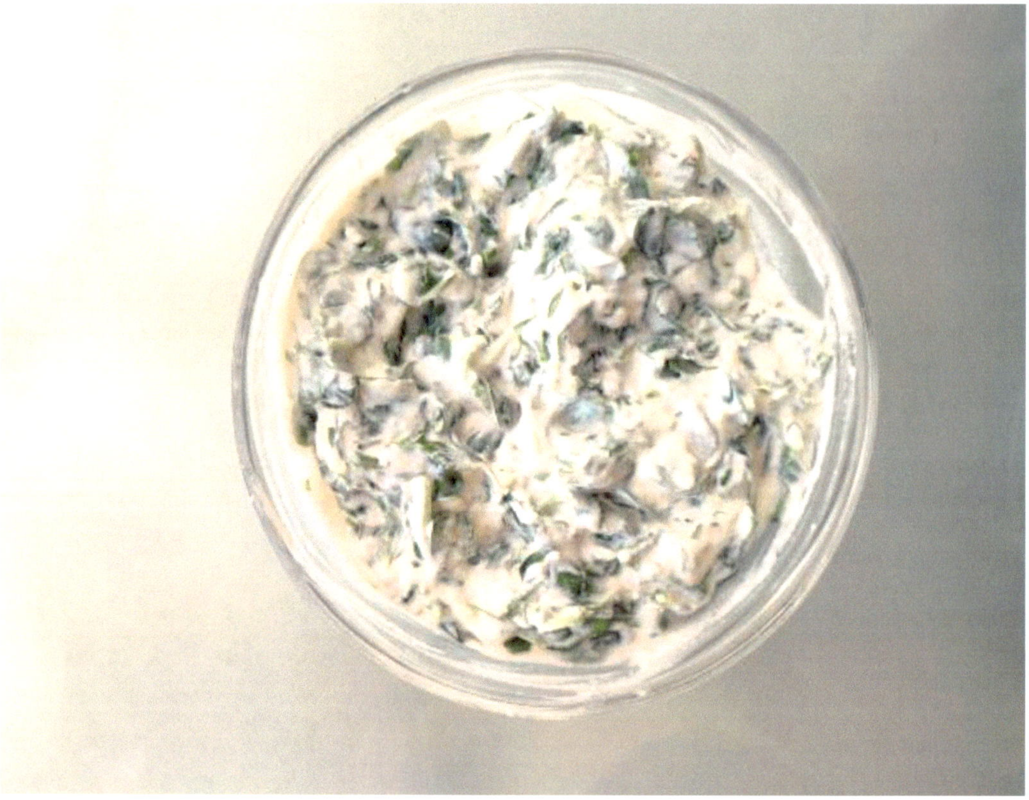

57. Garlic Parmesan Yogurt Dip

Prep.Time: 5 min

Cook Time: 0 min

Serving: 4

Ingredients:

- 1/2 cup Greek yogurt (low-fat or non-fat)
- 2 tablespoons grated Parmesan cheese
- 1 clove garlic, minced
- 1 tablespoon chopped fresh parsley
- 1 tablespoon lemon juice
- Salt and pepper to taste

Preparation:

1. In a mixing bowl, combine Greek yogurt, grated Parmesan cheese, minced garlic, chopped parsley, lemon juice, salt, and pepper.
2. Stir well until all ingredients are thoroughly combined.
3. Taste and adjust seasoning if necessary.
4. Serve immediately as a dip for vegetable sticks, pita chips, or as a spread for sandwiches or wraps.

Nutrient Facts (per serving):

- Calories: 60
- Carbohydrates: 2g
- Fat: 4g
- Protein: 4g

58. Sugar-Free Cranberry Relish

Prep.Time: 10 min | **Cook Time:** 5 min | **Serving:** 4

Ingredients:

- 1 cup fresh cranberries
- 1/4 cup water
- 2 tablespoons erythritol (or another sugar substitute)
- 1 tablespoon orange zest
- 1 tablespoon lemon juice
- Pinch of cinnamon (optional)

Preparation:

1. In a saucepan, combine fresh cranberries, water, erythritol, orange zest, lemon juice, and cinnamon (if using).
2. Cook over medium heat, stirring occasionally, until the cranberries burst and the mixture thickens slightly, about 5 minutes.
3. Remove from heat and let cool before serving.
4. Transfer to a glass jar or container with a lid.
5. Store in the refrigerator for up to one week.

Nutrient Facts (per serving):

- Calories: 30
- Carbohydrates: 8g
- Fat: 0g
- Protein: 0g

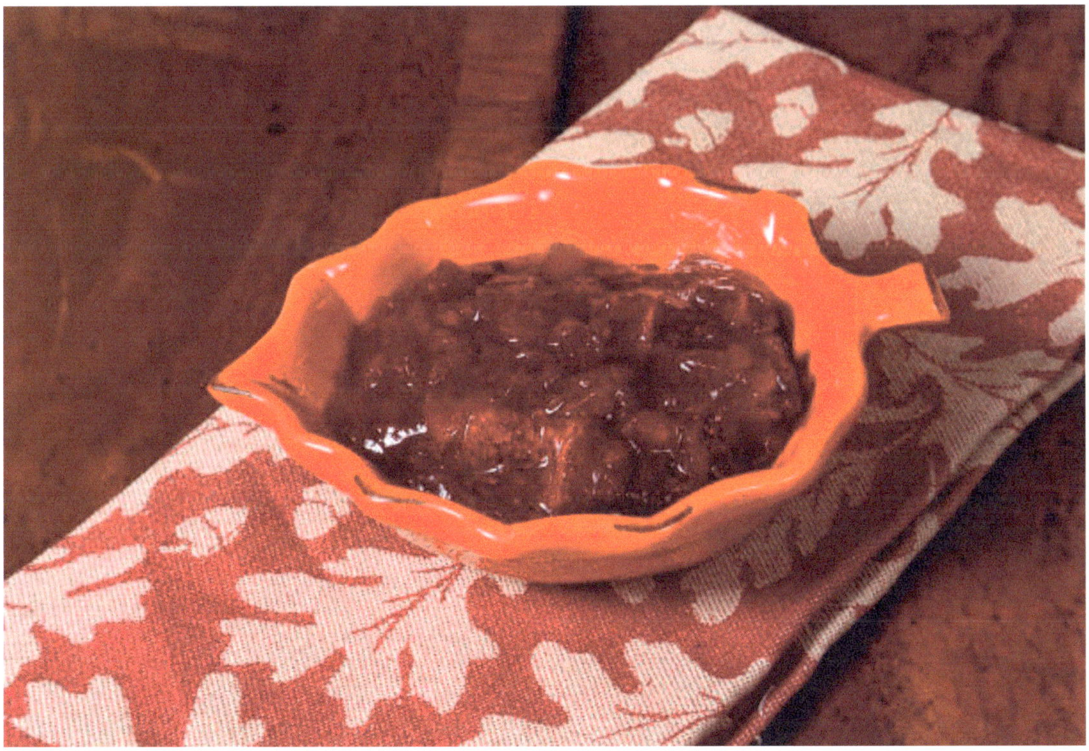

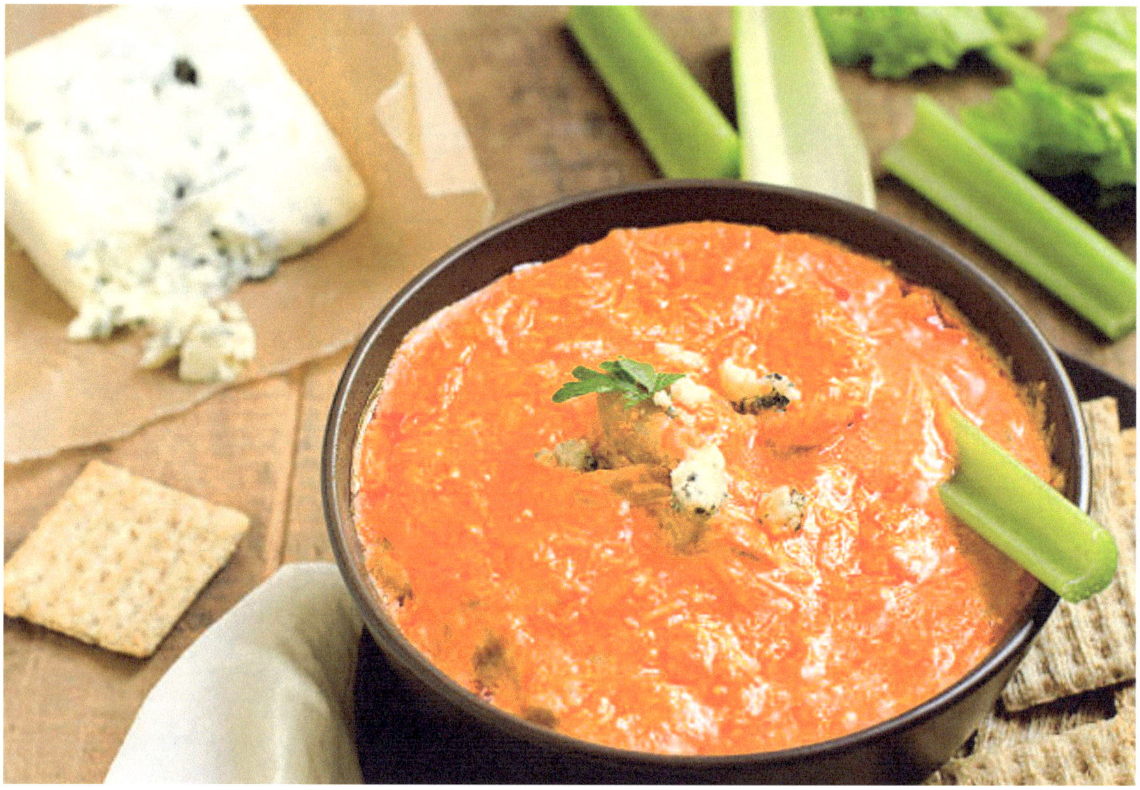

59. Thai Basil Peanut Dip

Prep.Time:	Cook Time:	Serving:
10 min	0 min	4

Ingredients:

- 1/4 cup creamy peanut butter
- 2 tablespoons coconut milk
- 1 tablespoon soy sauce (low-sodium, if preferred)
- 1 tablespoon lime juice
- 1 teaspoon minced garlic
- 1 teaspoon grated fresh ginger
- 1 tablespoon chopped fresh Thai basil leaves
- Pinch of red pepper flakes (optional)

Preparation:

1. In a small bowl, whisk together creamy peanut butter, coconut milk, soy sauce, lime juice, minced garlic, grated ginger, chopped Thai basil leaves, and red pepper flakes (if using) until smooth and creamy.
2. Taste and adjust seasoning if necessary.
3. Serve immediately as a dipping sauce for spring rolls, satay, or as a sauce for noodles or stir-fries.

Nutrient Facts (per serving):

- Calories: 80
- Carbohydrates: 4g
- Fat: 6g
- Protein: 3g

60. Baba Ganoush with Toasted Sesame Seeds

Prep.Time: 10 min

Cook Time: 30 min

Serving: 4

Ingredients:

- 2 medium eggplants
- 2 tablespoons tahini (sesame seed paste)
- 1 tablespoon lemon juice
- 1 clove garlic, minced
- 1 tablespoon extra virgin olive oil
- Salt and pepper to taste
- 1 tablespoon toasted sesame seeds (for garnish)
- Chopped fresh parsley (for garnish)

Preparation:

1. Preheat the oven to 400°F (200°C).
2. Prick the eggplants with a fork and place them on a baking sheet.
3. Roast in the preheated oven for 25-30 minutes, or until the eggplants are very soft and collapsed.
4. Remove from the oven and let cool slightly.
5. Cut the eggplants in half and scoop out the flesh into a bowl.
6. Add tahini, lemon juice, minced garlic, extra virgin olive oil, salt, and pepper to the bowl with the eggplant flesh.
7. Mash and mix everything together until well combined and smooth.
8. Taste and adjust seasoning if necessary.
9. Transfer the baba ganoush to a serving dish.
10. Garnish with toasted sesame seeds and chopped fresh parsley.
11. Serve with pita bread, vegetable sticks, or as a spread for sandwiches or wraps.

Nutrient Facts (per serving):

- Calories: 60
- Carbohydrates: 6g
- Fat: 4g
- Protein: 2g

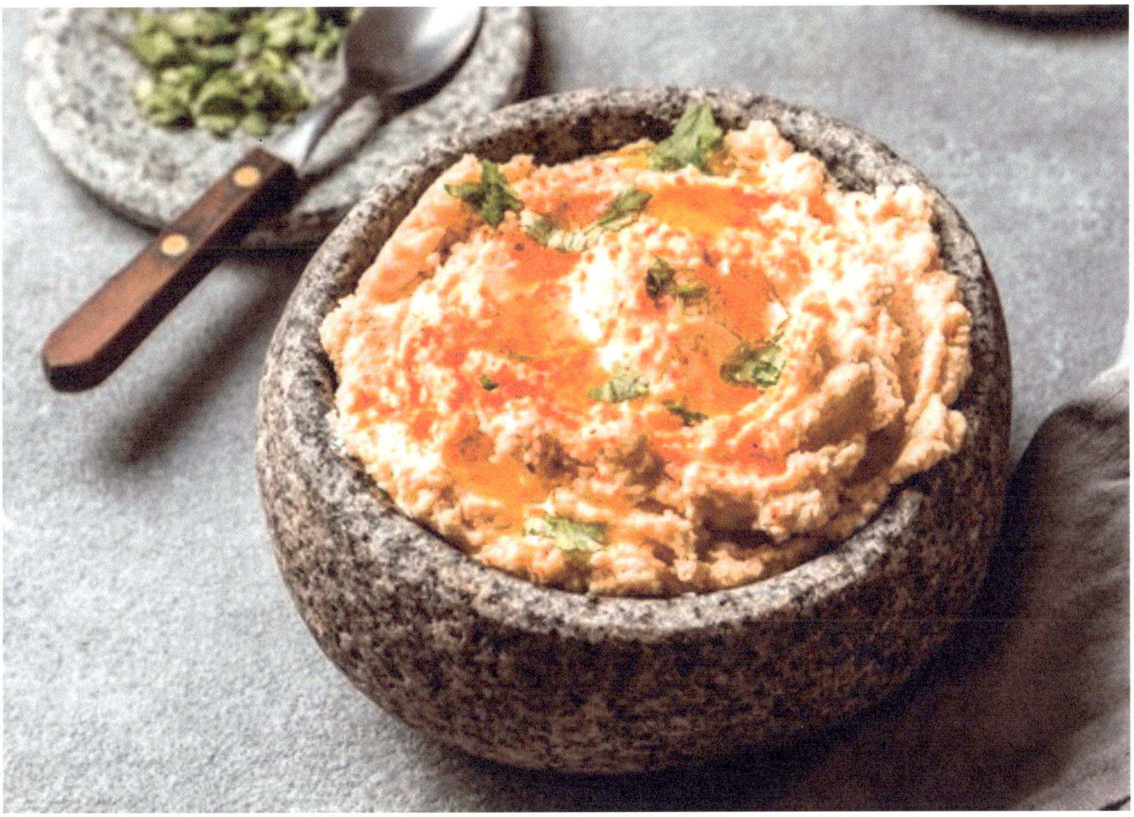

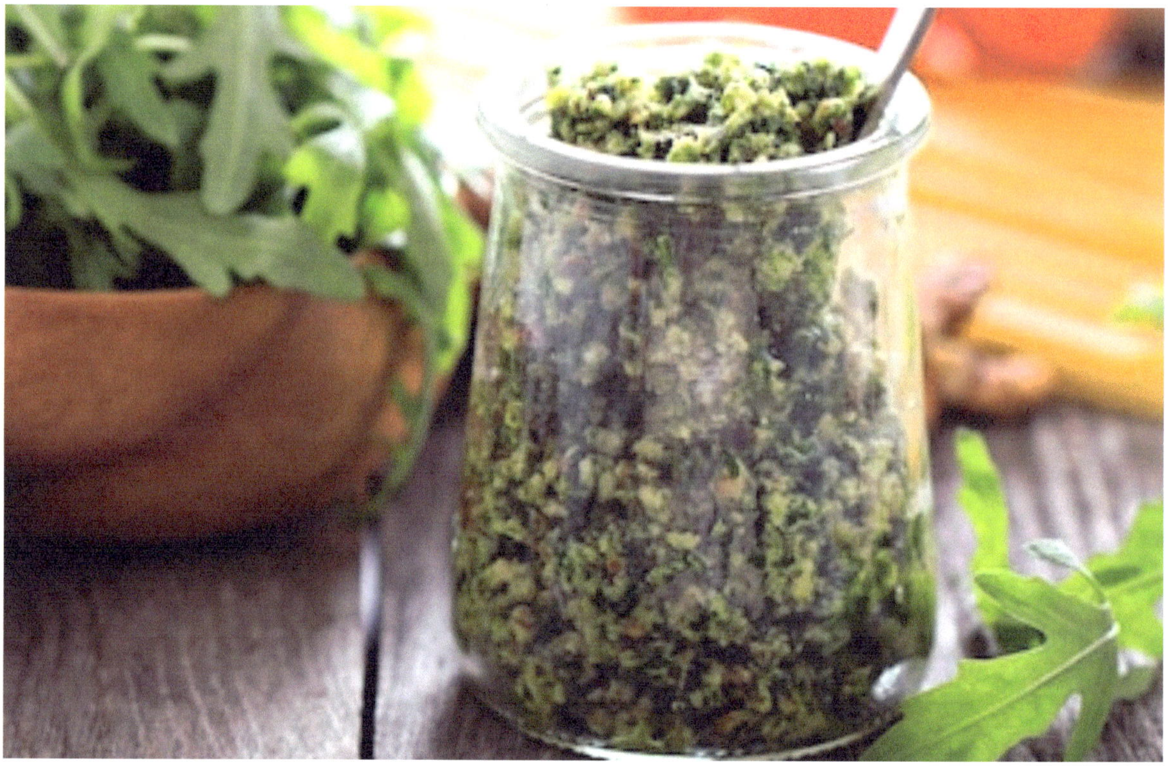

61. Chimichurri Sauce with Fresh Herbs

Prep.Time: 10 min

Cook Time: 0 min

Serving: 4

Ingredients:

- 1/2 cup fresh parsley leaves
- 1/4 cup fresh cilantro leaves
- 2 cloves garlic, minced
- 2 tablespoons red wine vinegar
- 1/4 cup extra virgin olive oil
- 1/2 teaspoon dried oregano
- 1/2 teaspoon dried thyme
- Salt and pepper to taste
- Pinch of red pepper flakes (optional)

Preparation:

1. In a food processor or blender, combine fresh parsley leaves, fresh cilantro leaves, minced garlic, red wine vinegar, extra virgin olive oil, dried oregano, dried thyme, salt, pepper, and red pepper flakes (if using).
2. Pulse until the herbs are finely chopped and the sauce is well blended but still slightly chunky.
3. Taste and adjust seasoning if necessary.
4. Transfer the chimichurri sauce to a serving bowl.
5. Serve immediately as a sauce for grilled meats, seafood, or vegetables.

Nutrient Facts (per serving):

- Calories: 70
- Carbohydrates: 2g
- Fat: 7g
- Protein: 1g

62. Creamy Horseradish Mustard Dressing

Prep.Time: 5 min | **Cook Time:** 0 min | **Serving:** 4

Ingredients:

- 1/4 cup Greek yogurt (low-fat or non-fat)
- 1 tablespoon prepared horseradish
- 1 tablespoon Dijon mustard
- 1 tablespoon lemon juice
- 1 teaspoon honey or maple syrup
- Salt and pepper to taste

Preparation:

1. In a small bowl, whisk together Greek yogurt, prepared horseradish, Dijon mustard, lemon juice, honey or maple syrup, salt, and pepper until smooth and creamy.
2. Taste and adjust seasoning if necessary.
3. Serve immediately over salads, roasted vegetables, or grilled meats.

Nutrient Facts (per serving):

- Calories: 50
- Carbohydrates: 1g
- Fat: 4g
- Protein: 2g

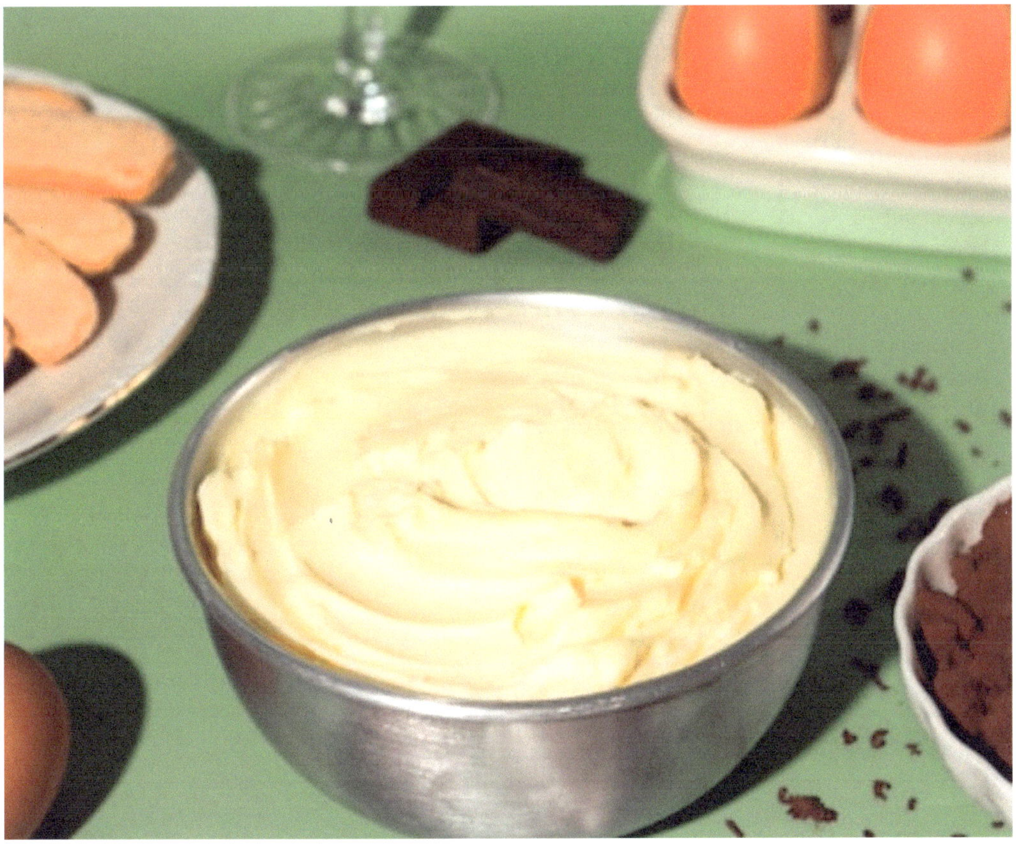

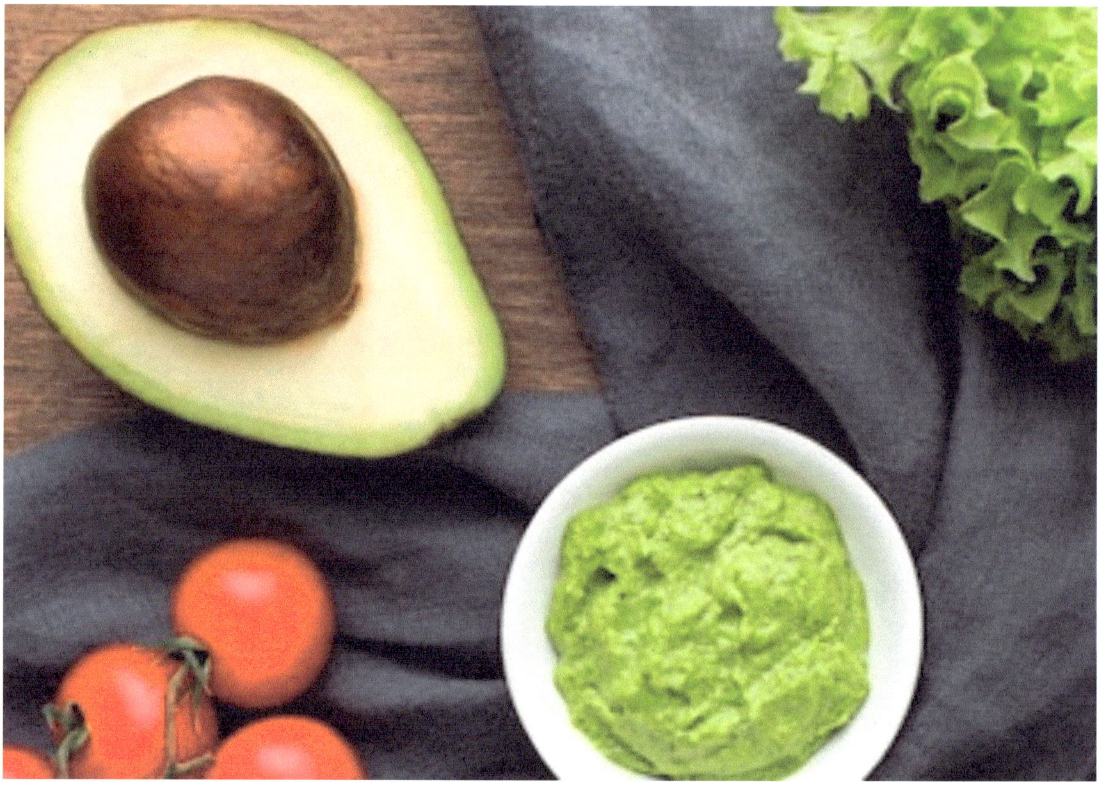

63. Tomatillo Avocado Salsa

Prep.Time: 15 min

Cook Time: 10 min

Serving: 4

Ingredients:

- 4 tomatillos, husked and washed
- 1 ripe avocado, peeled and diced
- 1/4 cup chopped fresh cilantro
- 1 jalapeño pepper, seeded and chopped
- 1/4 cup diced red onion
- 2 tablespoons lime juice
- Salt and pepper to taste

Preparation:

1. Preheat broiler to high.
2. Place the tomatillos on a baking sheet and broil for about 5-7 minutes, or until slightly charred and softened.
3. Remove from the oven and let cool slightly.
4. In a blender or food processor, combine the broiled tomatillos, diced avocado, chopped cilantro, chopped jalapeño pepper, diced red onion, and lime juice.
5. Pulse until the mixture reaches your desired consistency.
6. Season with salt and pepper according to taste.
7. Transfer the salsa to a serving bowl.
8. Serve with tortilla chips, tacos, grilled meats, or fish.

Nutrient Facts (per serving):

- Calories: 50
- Carbohydrates: 3g
- Fat: 4g
- Protein: 1g

64. Pomegranate Balsamic Vinaigrette

Prep.Time: 5 min | **Cook Time:** 0 min | **Serving:** 4

Ingredients:

- 1/4 cup pomegranate juice
- 2 tablespoons balsamic vinegar
- 2 tablespoons extra virgin olive oil
- 1 teaspoon Dijon mustard
- 1/2 teaspoon honey or maple syrup
- Salt and pepper to taste

Preparation:

1. In a small bowl, whisk together pomegranate juice, balsamic vinegar, extra virgin olive oil, Dijon mustard, honey or maple syrup, salt, and pepper until well combined.
2. Taste and adjust seasoning if necessary.
3. Serve immediately over salads, roasted vegetables, or grilled meats.

Nutrient Facts (per serving):

- Calories: 60
- Carbohydrates: 4g
- Fat: 4g
- Protein: 0g

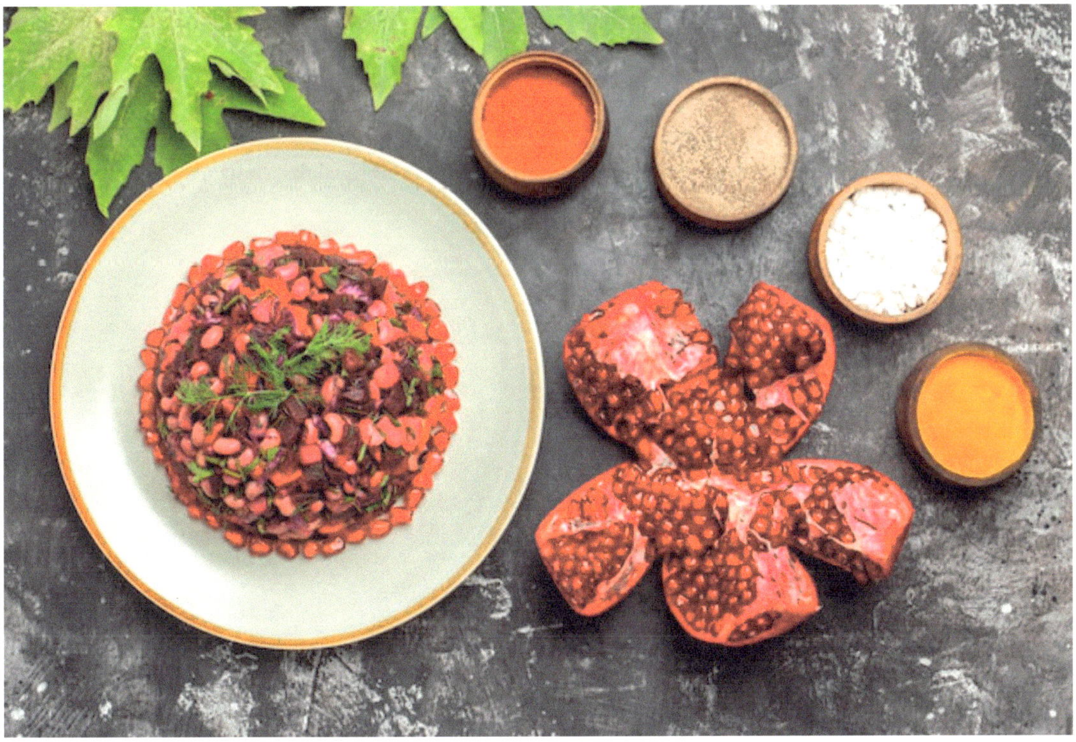

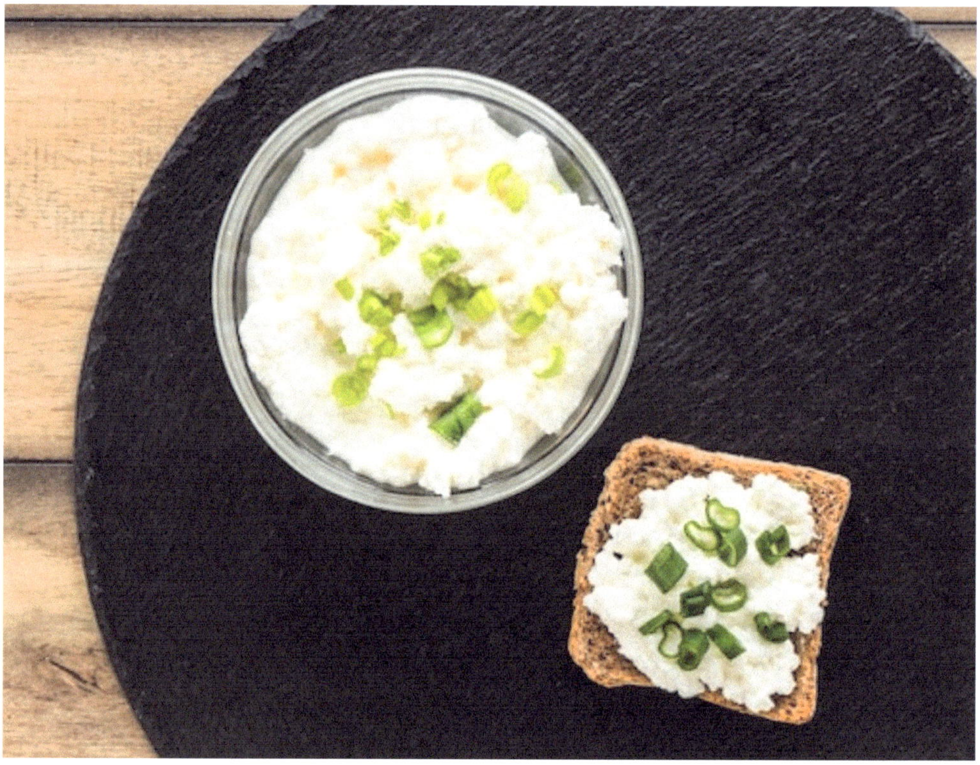

65. Greek Olive and Feta Dip

Prep.Time:	Cook Time:	Serving:
10 min	0 min	4

Ingredients:

- 1/2 cup crumbled feta cheese
- 1/4 cup Greek yogurt
- 1/4 cup chopped Kalamata olives
- 1 tablespoon chopped fresh parsley
- 1 tablespoon chopped fresh dill
- 1 clove garlic, minced
- 1 tablespoon lemon juice
- Black pepper to taste

Preparation:

1. In a mixing bowl, combine crumbled feta cheese, Greek yogurt, chopped Kalamata olives, chopped parsley, chopped dill, minced garlic, and lemon juice.
2. Mix well until all ingredients are thoroughly combined.
3. Season with black pepper according to taste.
4. Taste and adjust seasoning if necessary.
5. Serve chilled with pita bread, vegetable sticks, or as a spread for sandwiches or wraps.

Nutrient Facts (per serving):

- Calories: 70
- Carbohydrates: 2g
- Fat: 6g
- Protein: 2g

66. Harissa Yogurt Sauce

Prep.Time:	Cook Time:	Serving:
5 min	0 min	4

Ingredients:

- 1/2 cup Greek yogurt (low-fat or non-fat)
- 1 tablespoon harissa paste
- 1 tablespoon lemon juice
- 1 teaspoon maple syrup
- Salt to taste

Preparation:

1. In a small bowl, whisk together Greek yogurt, harissa paste, lemon juice, maple syrup, and salt until smooth.
2. Taste and adjust seasoning if necessary.
3. Serve immediately as a sauce for grilled meats, roasted vegetables, or as a dip for pita chips or vegetable sticks.

Nutrient Facts (per serving):

- Calories: 40
- Carbohydrates: 3g
- Fat: 2g
- Protein: 2g

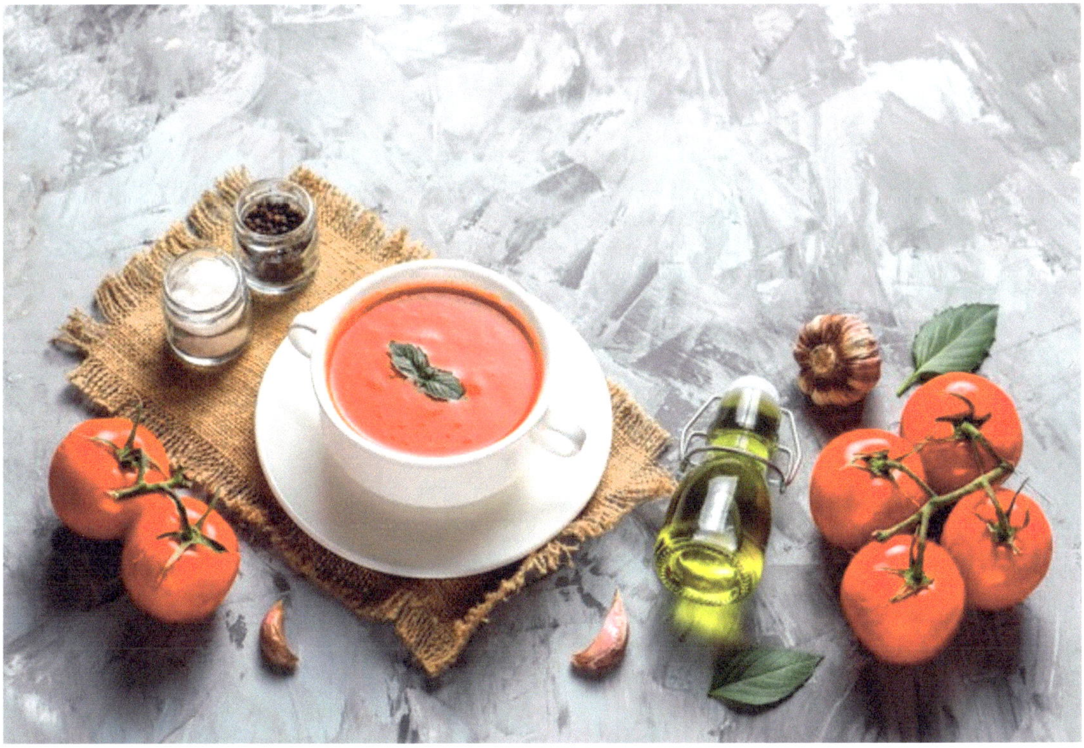

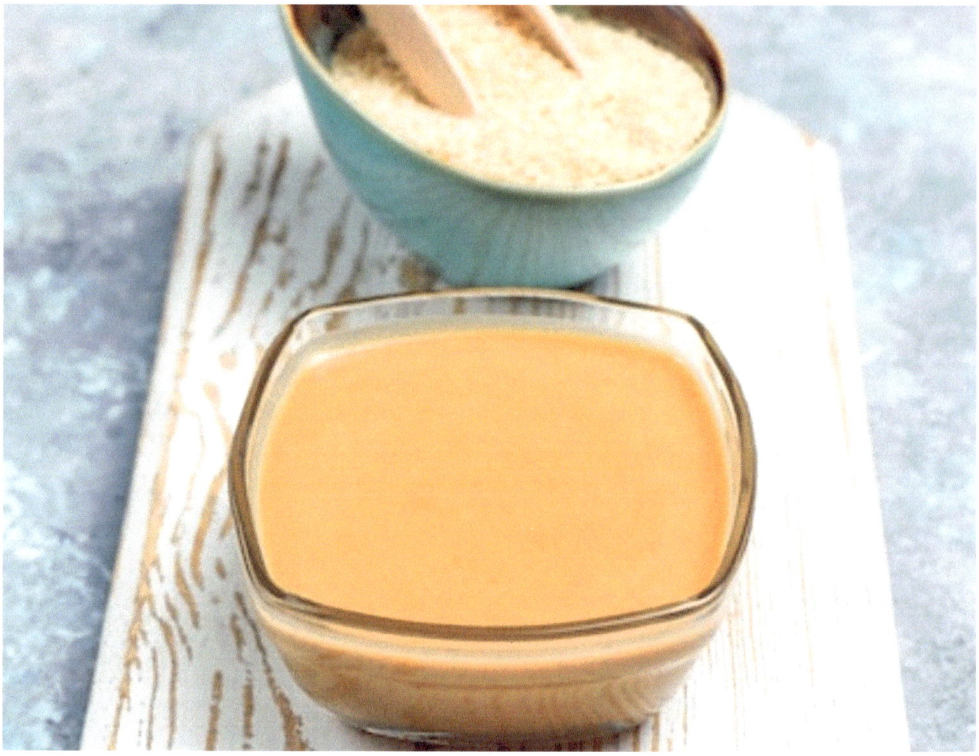

67. Sesame Almond Butter Sauce

Prep.Time: 5 min

Cook Time: 0 min

Serving: 4

Ingredients:

- 2 tablespoons almond butter
- 1 tablespoon sesame oil
- 1 tablespoon soy sauce (low-sodium, if preferred)
- 1 tablespoon rice vinegar
- 1 teaspoon maple syrup
- 1 teaspoon minced ginger
- 1 clove garlic, minced
- Water (as needed to thin out the sauce)
- Sesame seeds (for garnish)

Preparation:

1. In a small bowl, whisk together almond butter, sesame oil, soy sauce, rice vinegar, maple syrup, minced ginger, and minced garlic until well combined.
2. If the sauce is too thick, add water gradually until you reach your desired consistency.
3. Taste and adjust seasoning if necessary.
4. Serve immediately as a dipping sauce for spring rolls, dumplings, or as a sauce for noodles or stir-fries.
5. Garnish with sesame seeds before serving.

Nutrient Facts (per serving):

- Calories: 70
- Carbohydrates: 3g
- Fat: 6g
- Protein: 3g

68. Low-Sodium Artichoke Spinach Dip

Prep.Time: 15 min

Cook Time: 15 min

Serving: 4

Ingredients:

- 1 cup frozen chopped spinach, thawed and drained
- 1 cup canned artichoke hearts, drained and chopped
- 1/2 cup Greek yogurt (low-fat or non-fat)
- 1/4 cup grated Parmesan cheese
- 1/4 cup mayonnaise (low-fat or olive oil-based)
- 2 cloves garlic, minced
- 1/2 teaspoon onion powder
- Salt and pepper to taste

Preparation:

1. Preheat the oven to 375°F (190°C).
2. In a mixing bowl, combine chopped spinach, chopped artichoke hearts, Greek yogurt, grated Parmesan cheese, mayonnaise, minced garlic, onion powder, salt, and pepper.
3. Mix well until all ingredients are thoroughly combined.
4. Transfer the mixture to an oven-safe baking dish.
5. Bake in the preheated oven for about 15 minutes, or until the dip is hot and bubbly.
6. Remove from the oven and let cool slightly before serving.
7. Serve with whole grain crackers, vegetable sticks, or toasted bread.

Nutrient Facts (per serving):

- Calories: 80
- Carbohydrates: 4g
- Fat: 6g
- Protein: 3g

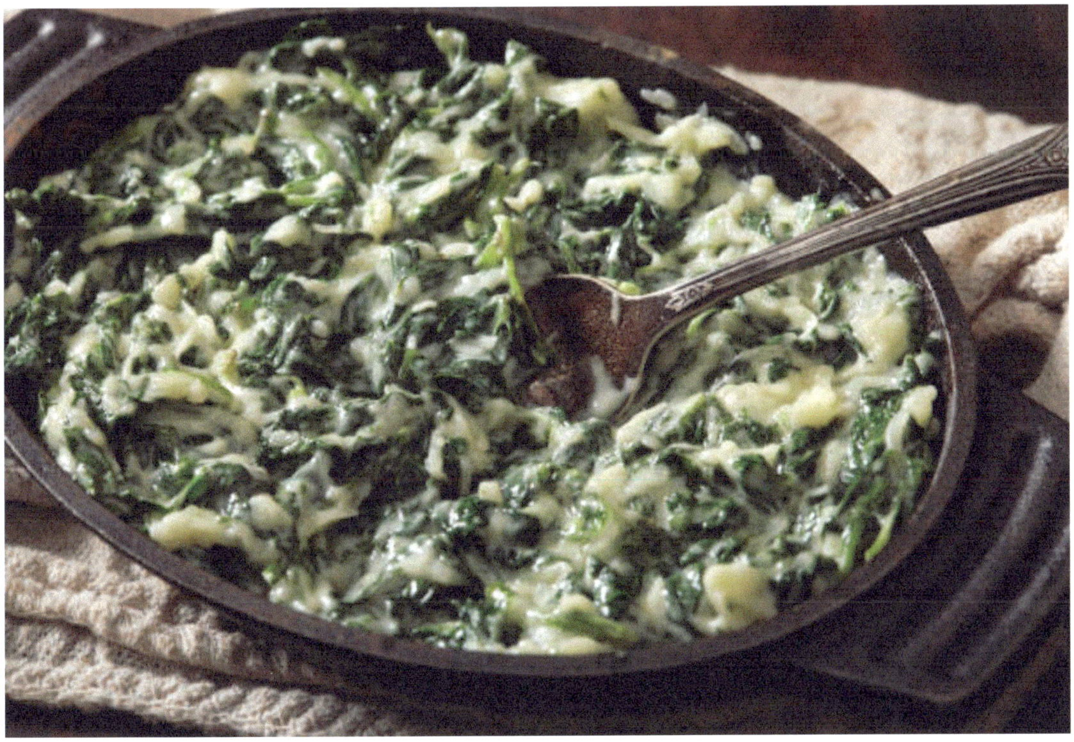

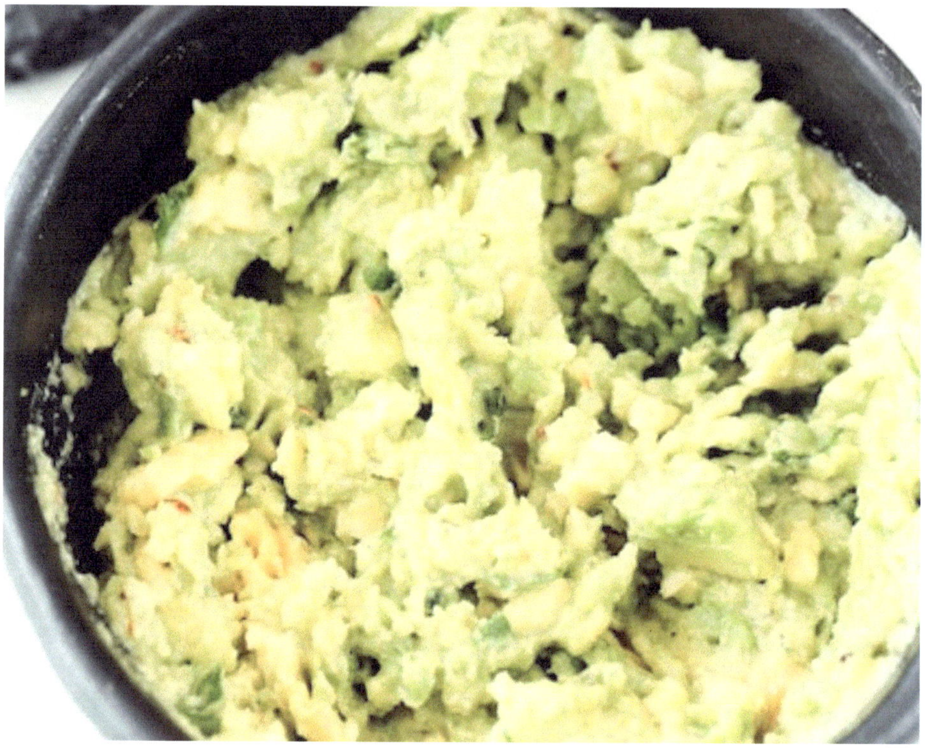

69. Cilantro Lime Cashew Cream

Prep.Time:	Cook Time:	Serving:
10 min	0 min	4

Ingredients:

- 1 cup raw cashews, soaked in water for at least 2 hours, drained
- 1/4 cup water
- 2 tablespoons lime juice
- 1/4 cup chopped fresh cilantro
- 1 clove garlic, minced
- Salt and pepper to taste

Preparation:

1. In a blender or food processor, combine soaked cashews, water, lime juice, chopped cilantro, minced garlic, salt, and pepper.
2. Blend until smooth and creamy, adding more water if necessary to reach your desired consistency.
3. Taste and adjust seasoning if necessary.
4. Serve immediately as a topping for tacos, burrito bowls, or as a dip for vegetable sticks.

Nutrient Facts (per serving):

- Calories: 90
- Carbohydrates: 5g
- Fat: 7g
- Protein: 3g

70. Tomato Basil Yogurt Dressing

Prep.Time: 10 min | **Cook Time:** 0 min | **Serving:** 4

Ingredients:

- 1/2 cup Greek yogurt (low-fat or non-fat)
- 1/4 cup chopped fresh basil
- 2 tablespoons chopped sun-dried tomatoes (packed in oil)
- 1 tablespoon lemon juice
- 1 clove garlic, minced
- Salt and pepper to taste

Preparation:

1. In a small bowl, whisk together Greek yogurt, chopped basil, chopped sun-dried tomatoes, lemon juice, minced garlic, salt, and pepper until well combined.
2. Taste and adjust seasoning if necessary.
3. Serve immediately over salads, grilled vegetables, or as a dip for vegetable sticks.

Nutrient Facts (per serving):

- Calories: 60
- Carbohydrates: 3g
- Fat: 4g
- Protein: 3g

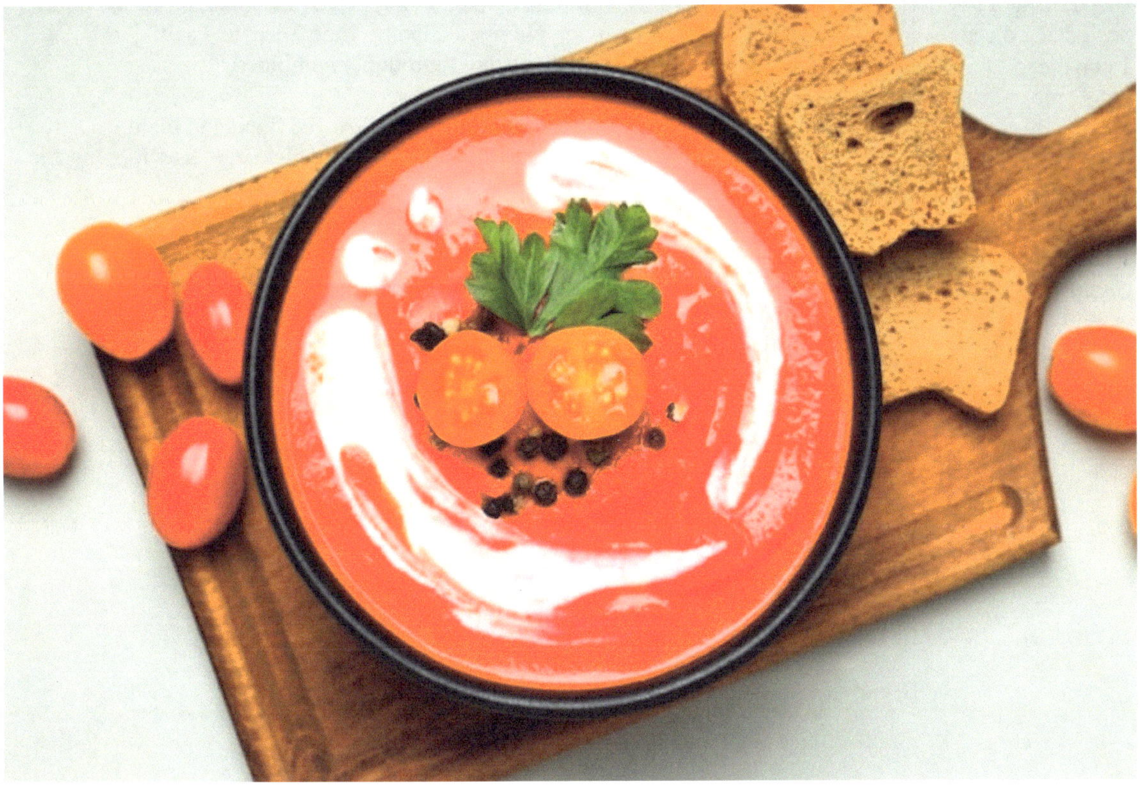

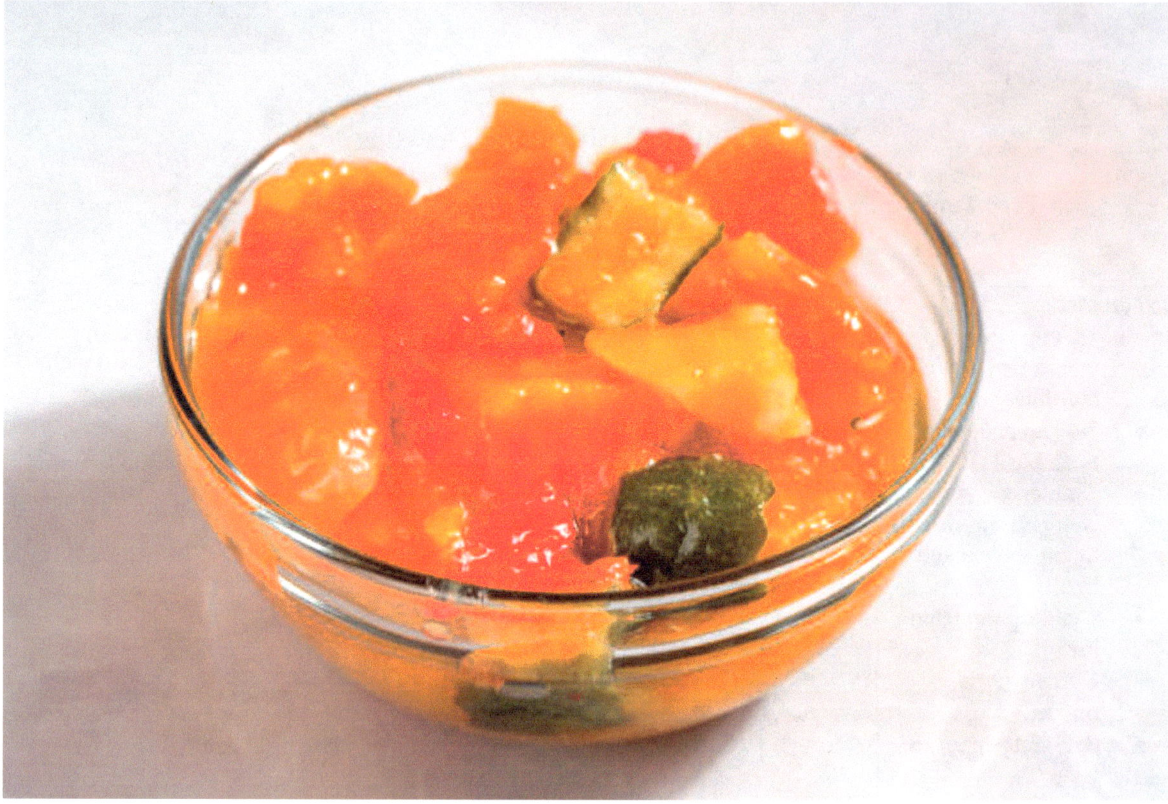

71. Mango Pineapple Salsa

Prep.Time:	Cook Time:	Serving:
15 min	0 min	4

Ingredients:

- 1 ripe mango, peeled and diced
- 1 cup diced pineapple
- 1/4 cup diced red onion
- 1 jalapeño pepper, seeded and minced
- 2 tablespoons chopped fresh cilantro
- 1 tablespoon lime juice
- Salt to taste

Preparation:

1. In a mixing bowl, combine diced mango, diced pineapple, diced red onion, minced jalapeño pepper, chopped cilantro, lime juice, and salt.
2. Mix well until all ingredients are thoroughly combined.
3. Taste and adjust seasoning if necessary.
4. Let the salsa sit for about 10 minutes to allow the flavors to meld.
5. Serve chilled with tortilla chips, grilled fish or chicken, or as a topping for tacos.

Nutrient Facts (per serving):

- Calories: 60
- Carbohydrates: 15g
- Fat: 0g
- Protein: 1g

72. Roasted Red Pepper and Walnut Spread

Prep.Time: 15 min | **Cook Time:** 20 min | **Serving:** 4

Ingredients:

- 2 large red bell peppers
- 1/4 cup walnuts
- 2 tablespoons extra virgin olive oil
- 1 clove garlic, minced
- 1 tablespoon lemon juice
- Salt and pepper to taste

Preparation:

1. Preheat the broiler to high.
2. Place the whole red bell peppers on a baking sheet and broil, turning occasionally, until the skins are charred and blistered, about 10-15 minutes.
3. Remove the peppers from the oven and transfer them to a bowl. Cover with plastic wrap and let them steam for about 10 minutes.
4. Once cooled, peel off the skins, remove the seeds and stems, and roughly chop the flesh.
5. In a dry skillet, toast the walnuts over medium heat until fragrant, about 5 minutes.
6. In a food processor, combine the roasted red peppers, toasted walnuts, extra virgin olive oil, minced garlic, lemon juice, salt, and pepper.
7. Pulse until the mixture is smooth and well blended.
8. Taste and adjust seasoning if necessary.
9. Transfer the spread to a serving bowl.
10. Serve with crackers, bread, or as a spread for sandwiches or wraps.

Nutrient Facts (per serving):

- Calories: 90
- Carbohydrates: 3g
- Fat: 8g
- Protein: 2g

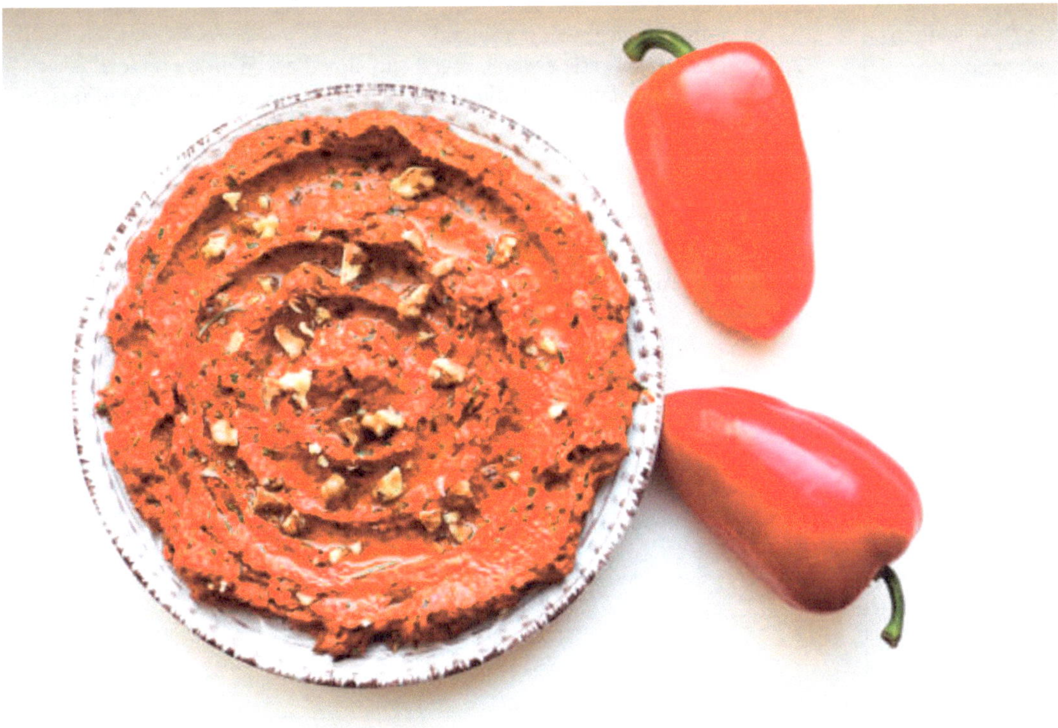

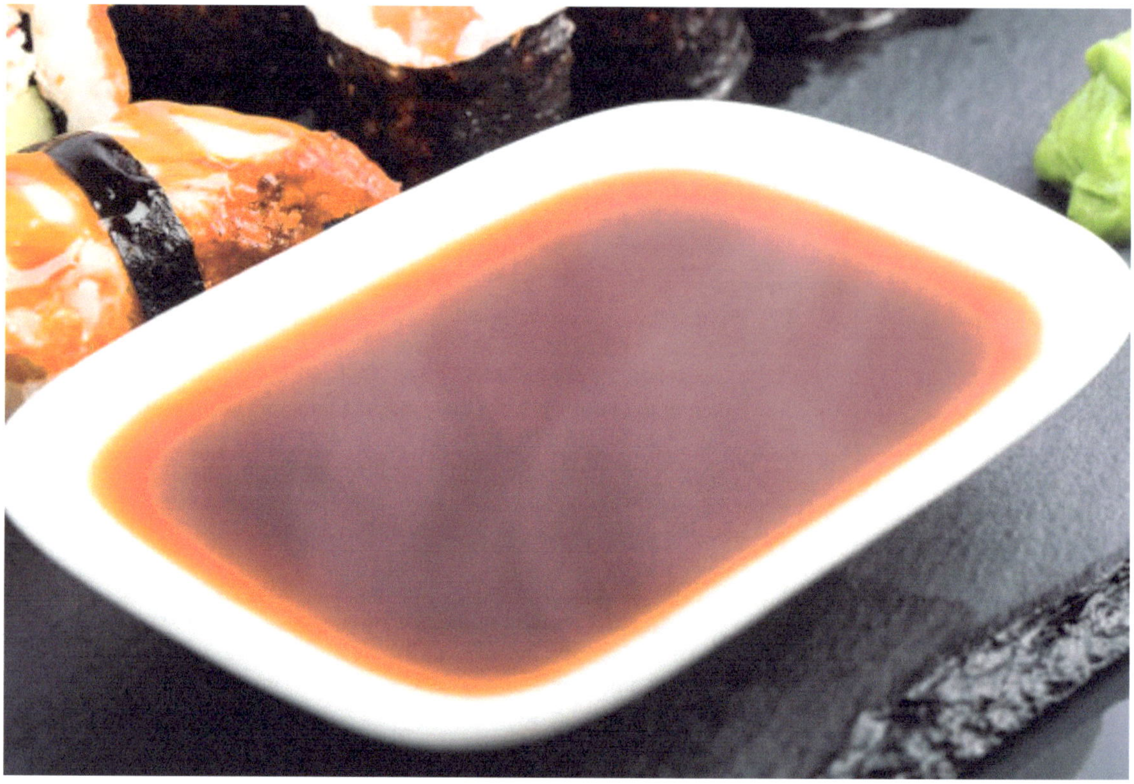

73. Soy Wasabi Dipping Sauce

Prep.Time: 5 min | **Cook Time:** 0 min | **Serving:** 4

Ingredients:

- 2 tablespoons soy sauce (low-sodium)
- 1 tablespoon rice vinegar
- 1 teaspoon wasabi paste
- 1 teaspoon sesame oil
- 1 teaspoon sesame seeds (optional)
- 1 green onion, thinly sliced (optional)

Preparation:

1. In a small bowl, whisk together soy sauce, rice vinegar, wasabi paste, and sesame oil until well combined.
2. If desired, sprinkle sesame seeds and sliced green onion on top.
3. Serve immediately as a dipping sauce for sushi, sashimi, dumplings, or grilled meats and vegetables.

Nutrient Facts (per serving):

- Calories: 30
- Carbohydrates: 2g
- Fat: 2g
- Protein: 1g

74. Cucumber and Mint Raita

Prep.Time: 10 min

Cook Time: 0 min

Serving: 4

Ingredients:

- 1 cup Greek yogurt (low-fat or non-fat)
- 1/2 cucumber, grated and excess moisture squeezed out
- 2 tablespoons chopped fresh mint leaves
- 1/2 teaspoon cumin powder
- Salt to taste

Preparation:

1. In a mixing bowl, combine Greek yogurt, grated cucumber, chopped mint leaves, cumin powder, and salt.
2. Mix well until all ingredients are thoroughly combined.
3. Taste and adjust seasoning if necessary.
4. Serve chilled as a side dish with Indian meals, or as a refreshing dip for naan bread, kebabs, or samosas.

Nutrient Facts (per serving):

- Calories: 40
- Carbohydrates: 3g
- Fat: 3g
- Protein: 2g

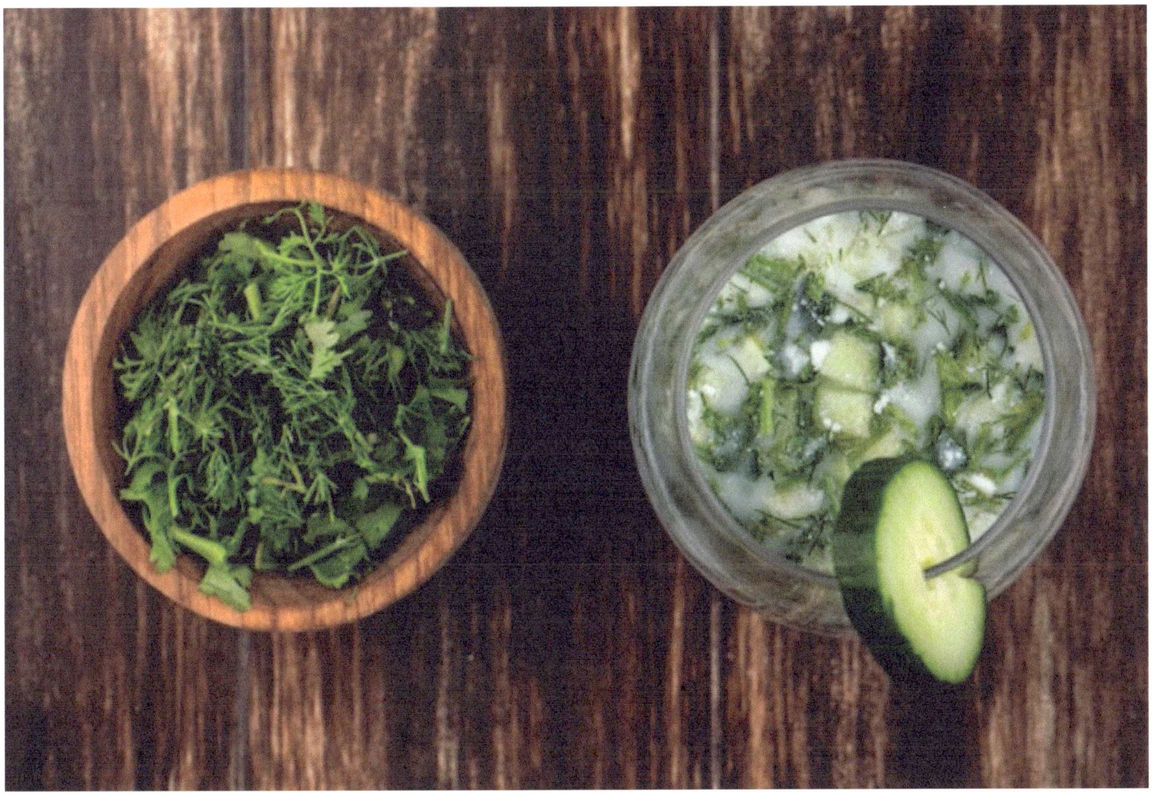

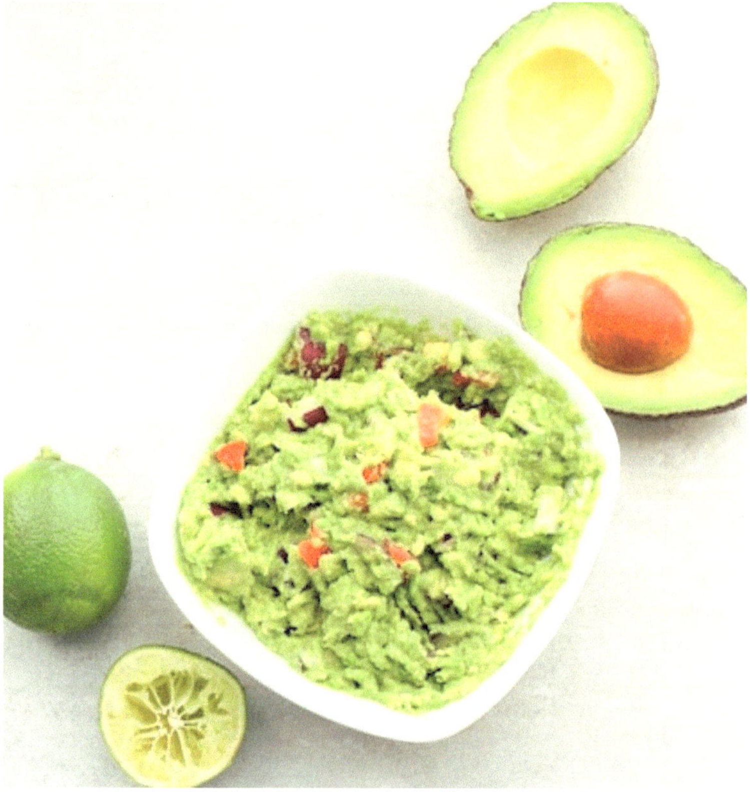

75. Avocado Basil Pesto

Prep.Time:	Cook Time:	Serving:
10 min	0 min	4

Ingredients:

- 1 ripe avocado, peeled and pitted
- 1 cup fresh basil leaves
- 1/4 cup pine nuts or walnuts
- 2 tablespoons grated Parmesan cheese
- 1 clove garlic, minced
- 1 tablespoon lemon juice
- 2 tablespoons extra virgin olive oil
- Salt and pepper to taste

Preparation:

1. In a food processor, combine ripe avocado, fresh basil leaves, pine nuts or walnuts, grated Parmesan cheese, minced garlic, lemon juice, extra virgin olive oil, salt, and pepper.
2. Pulse until the mixture is smooth and well blended, scraping down the sides as needed.
3. Taste and adjust seasoning if necessary.
4. Serve immediately tossed with cooked pasta, as a spread for sandwiches or wraps, or as a dip for vegetable sticks or crackers.

Nutrient Facts (per serving):

- Calories: 120
- Carbohydrates: 3g
- Fat: 11g
- Protein: 2g

76. Cilantro Lime Avocado Yogurt Sauce

Prep.Time: 5 min | **Cook Time:** 0 min | **Serving:** 4

Ingredients:

- 1 ripe avocado, peeled and pitted
- 1/4 cup Greek yogurt (low-fat or non-fat)
- 1/4 cup chopped fresh cilantro
- 1 tablespoon lime juice
- 1 clove garlic, minced
- Salt and pepper to taste

Preparation:

1. In a blender or food processor, combine ripe avocado, Greek yogurt, chopped cilantro, lime juice, minced garlic, salt, and pepper.
2. Blend until smooth and creamy.
3. Taste and adjust seasoning if necessary.
4. Serve immediately as a sauce for tacos, burrito bowls, grilled meats, or as a dip for tortilla chips or vegetable sticks.

Nutrient Facts (per serving):

- Calories: 70
- Carbohydrates: 4g
- Fat: 5g
- Protein: 2g

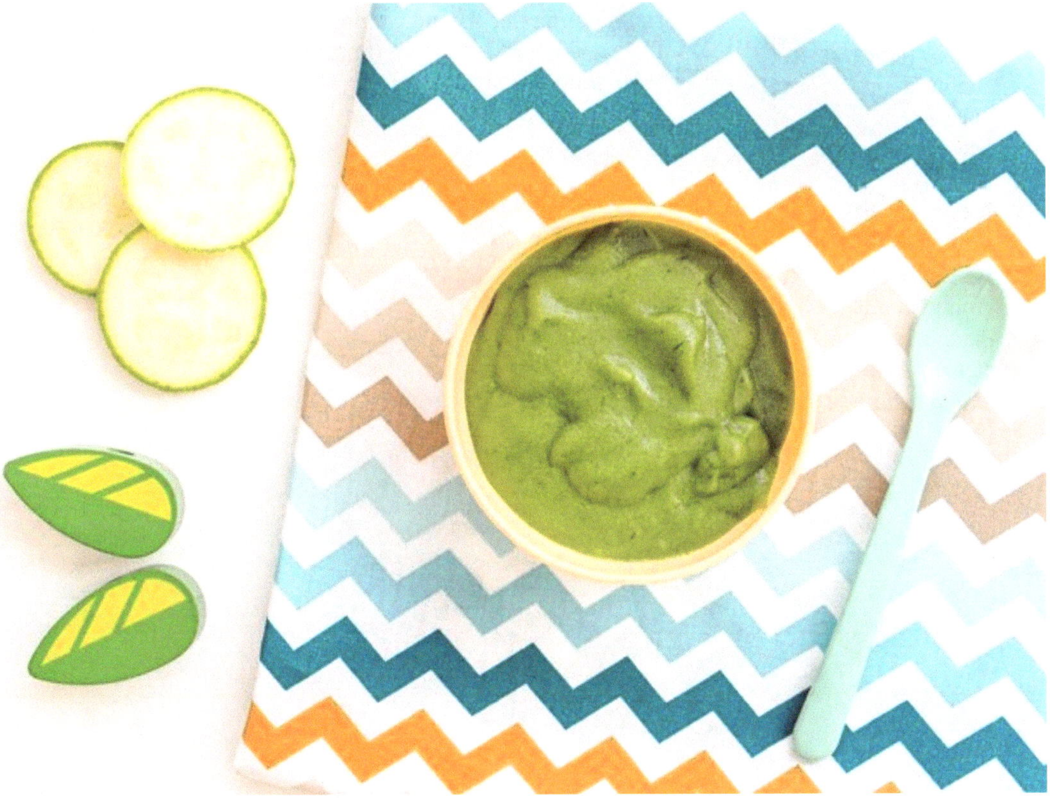

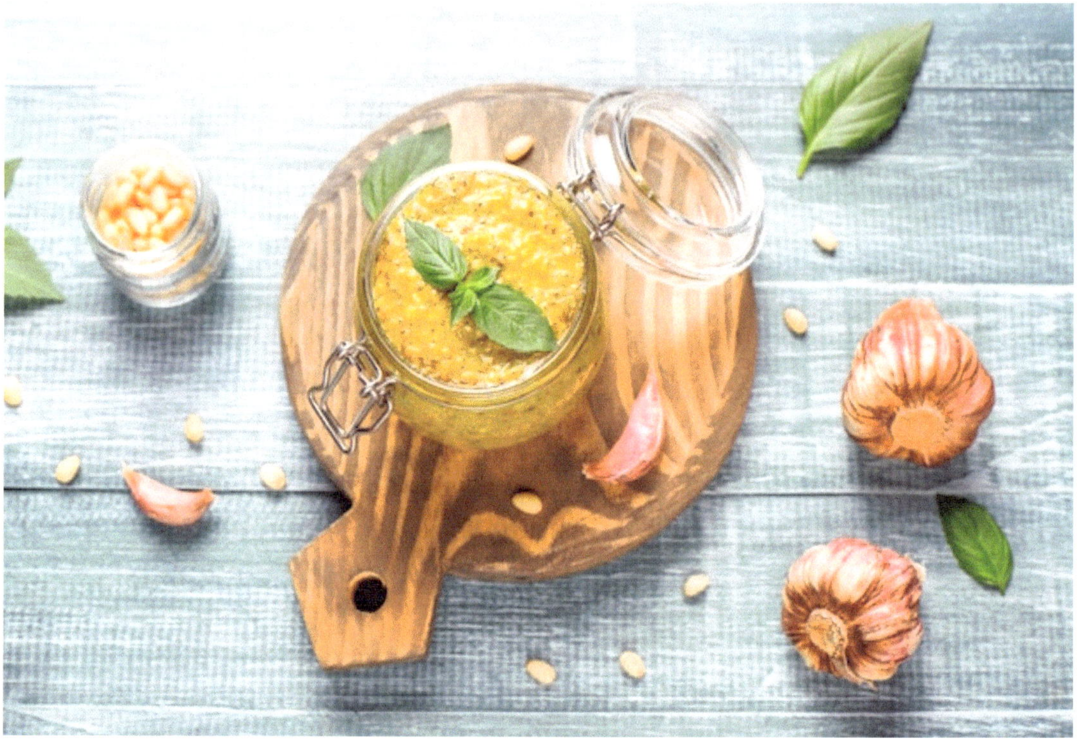

77. Turmeric Tahini Dressing

Prep.Time: 5 min | **Cook Time:** 0 min | **Serving:** 4

Ingredients:

- 2 tablespoons tahini (sesame seed paste)
- 2 tablespoons water
- 1 tablespoon lemon juice
- 1 teaspoon maple syrup
- 1/2 teaspoon ground turmeric
- 1/4 teaspoon ground cumin
- Pinch of cayenne pepper
- Salt to taste

Preparation:

1. In a small bowl, whisk together tahini, water, lemon juice, maple syrup, ground turmeric, ground cumin, cayenne pepper, and salt until smooth.
2. Taste and adjust seasoning if necessary.
3. Serve immediately over salads, roasted vegetables, or grilled meats.

Nutrient Facts (per serving):

- Calories: 70
- Carbohydrates: 3g
- Fat: 6g
- Protein: 2g

78. Roasted Vegetable Salsa

Prep.Time: 15 min | **Cook Time:** 25 min | **Serving:** 4

Ingredients:

- 1 cup diced mixed roasted vegetables (such as bell peppers, zucchini, onions, and corn)
- 1 medium tomato, diced
- 1/4 cup diced red onion
- 2 tablespoons chopped fresh cilantro
- 1 tablespoon lime juice
- Salt and pepper to taste

Preparation:

1. Preheat the oven to 400°F (200°C).
2. Toss the diced mixed vegetables with a drizzle of olive oil, salt, and pepper.
3. Spread the vegetables on a baking sheet and roast in the preheated oven for about 20-25 minutes, or until tender and slightly caramelized.
4. Remove from the oven and let cool slightly.
5. In a mixing bowl, combine the roasted vegetables, diced tomato, diced red onion, chopped cilantro, and lime juice.
6. Season with salt and pepper according to taste.
7. Mix well until all ingredients are combined.
8. Serve chilled or at room temperature with tortilla chips, grilled meats, or as a topping for tacos or burrito bowls.

Nutrient Facts (per serving):

- Calories: 35
- Carbohydrates: 6g
- Fat: 1g
- Protein: 1g

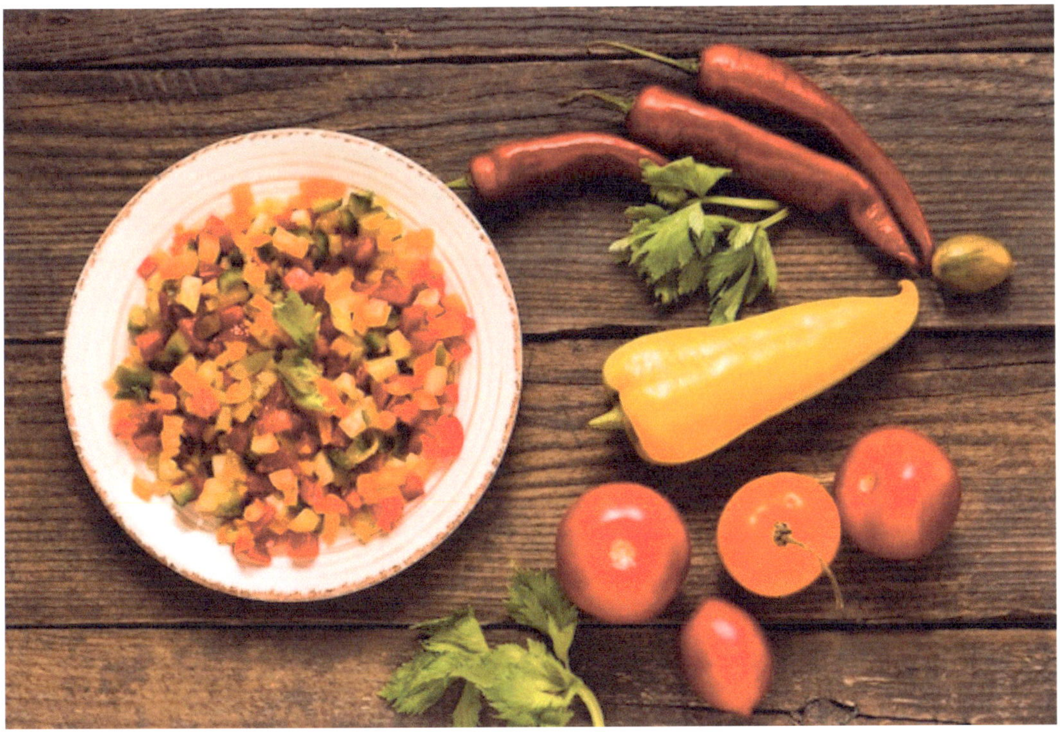

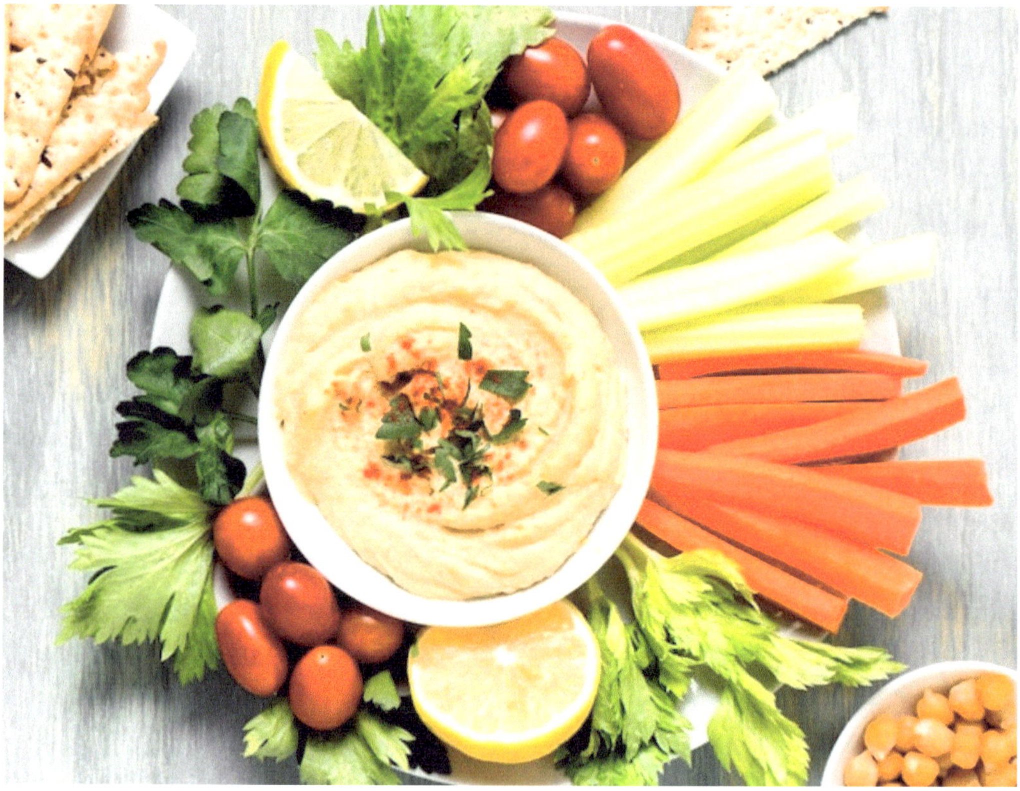

79. Lemon Herb Hummus

Prep.Time: 10 min

Cook Time: 0 min

Serving: 4

Ingredients:

- 1 can (15 ounces) chickpeas (garbanzo beans), drained and rinsed
- 2 tablespoons tahini (sesame seed paste)
- 2 tablespoons lemon juice
- 1 clove garlic, minced
- 1 tablespoon chopped fresh parsley
- 1 tablespoon chopped fresh dill
- 2 tablespoons extra virgin olive oil
- Salt and pepper to taste
- Water (as needed to adjust consistency)

Preparation:

1. In a food processor, combine chickpeas, tahini, lemon juice, minced garlic, chopped parsley, chopped dill, extra virgin olive oil, salt, and pepper.
2. Pulse until the mixture becomes coarse.
3. With the food processor running, drizzle in water, one tablespoon at a time, until the hummus reaches your desired consistency.
4. Continue to process until the hummus is smooth and creamy.
5. Taste and adjust seasoning if necessary.
6. Serve immediately or refrigerate until ready to serve.
7. Garnish with a drizzle of olive oil and a sprinkle of chopped fresh herbs before serving, if desired.

Nutrient Facts (per serving):

- Calories: 70
- Carbohydrates: 8g
- Fat: 3g
- Protein: 3g

80. Soy Sesame Ginger Dipping Sauce

Prep.Time: 5 min | **Cook Time:** 0 min | **Serving:** 4

Ingredients:

- 2 tablespoons soy sauce (low-sodium)
- 1 tablespoon rice vinegar
- 1 teaspoon sesame oil
- 1 teaspoon grated fresh ginger
- 1 teaspoon sesame seeds
- 1 green onion, thinly sliced (optional)

Preparation:

1. In a small bowl, whisk together soy sauce, rice vinegar, sesame oil, grated ginger, and sesame seeds until well combined.
2. If desired, garnish with thinly sliced green onion.
3. Serve immediately as a dipping sauce for sushi, spring rolls, dumplings, or grilled meats and vegetables.

Nutrient Facts (per serving):

- Calories: 40
- Carbohydrates: 3g
- Fat: 2g
- Protein: 2g

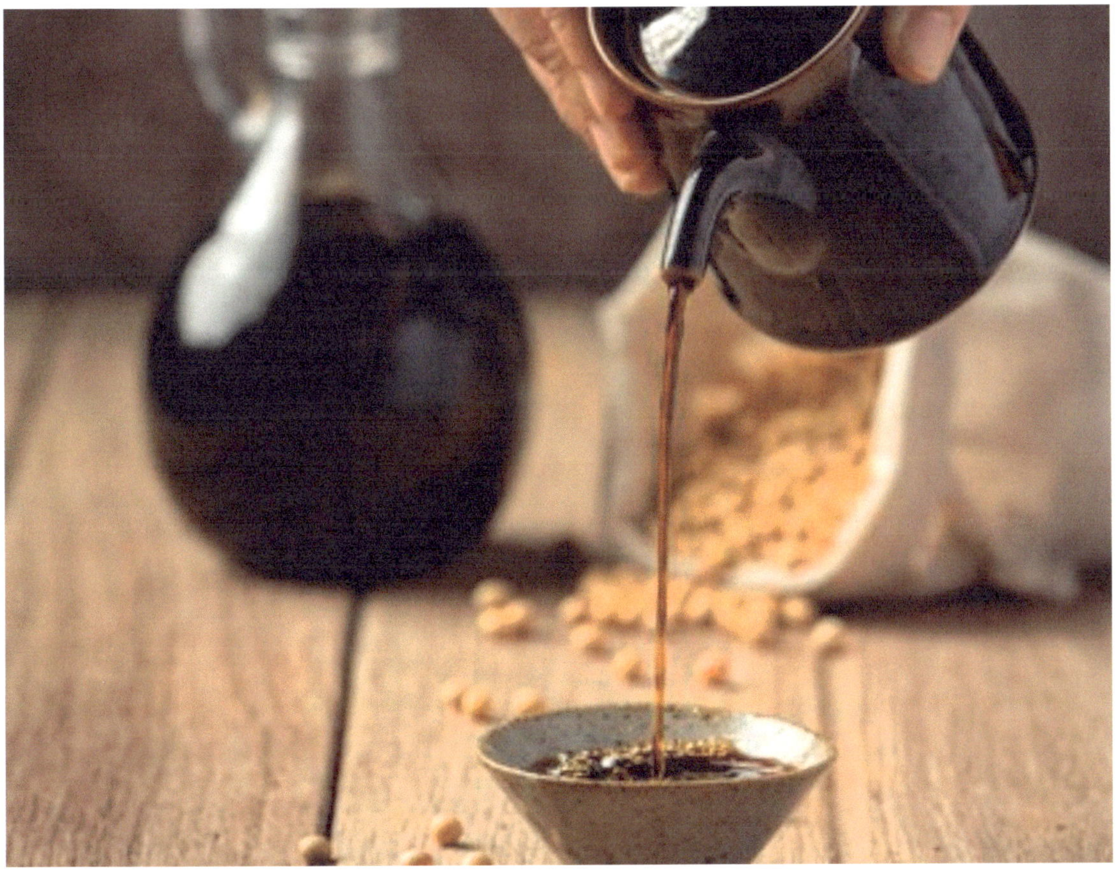

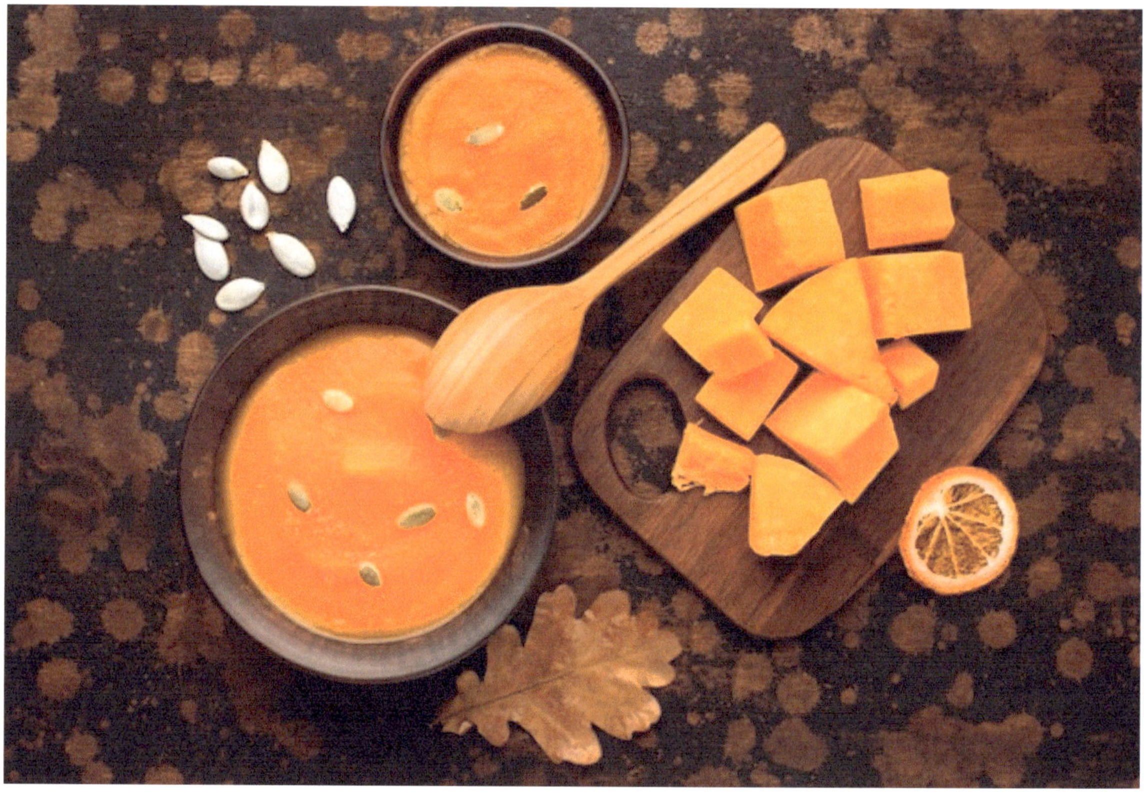

81. Spicy Mango Salsa

Prep.Time: 10 min | **Cook Time:** 0 min | **Serving:** 4

Ingredients:

- 1 ripe mango, peeled and diced
- 1/2 cup diced red bell pepper
- 2 tablespoons diced red onion
- 1 jalapeño pepper, seeded and minced
- 2 tablespoons chopped fresh cilantro
- 1 tablespoon lime juice
- Salt to taste

Preparation:

1. In a mixing bowl, combine diced mango, diced red bell pepper, diced red onion, minced jalapeño pepper, chopped cilantro, lime juice, and salt.
2. Mix well until all ingredients are thoroughly combined.
3. Taste and adjust seasoning if necessary.
4. Let the salsa sit for about 10 minutes to allow the flavors to meld.
5. Serve chilled with tortilla chips, grilled fish or chicken, or as a topping for tacos.

Nutrient Facts (per serving):

- Calories: 45
- Carbohydrates: 10g
- Fat: 0g
- Protein: 1g

82. Creamy Garlic Dill Yogurt Dip

Prep.Time: 10 min | **Cook Time:** 0 min | **Serving:** 4

Ingredients:

- 1 cup Greek yogurt (low-fat or non-fat)
- 1 clove garlic, minced
- 1 tablespoon chopped fresh dill
- 1 tablespoon lemon juice
- Salt and pepper to taste

Preparation:

1. In a mixing bowl, combine Greek yogurt, minced garlic, chopped fresh dill, lemon juice, salt, and pepper.
2. Mix well until all ingredients are thoroughly combined.
3. Taste and adjust seasoning if necessary.
4. Serve chilled as a dip for vegetable sticks, pita chips, or as a spread for sandwiches and wraps.

Nutrient Facts (per serving):

- Calories: 50
- Carbohydrates: 4g
- Fat: 2g
- Protein: 3g

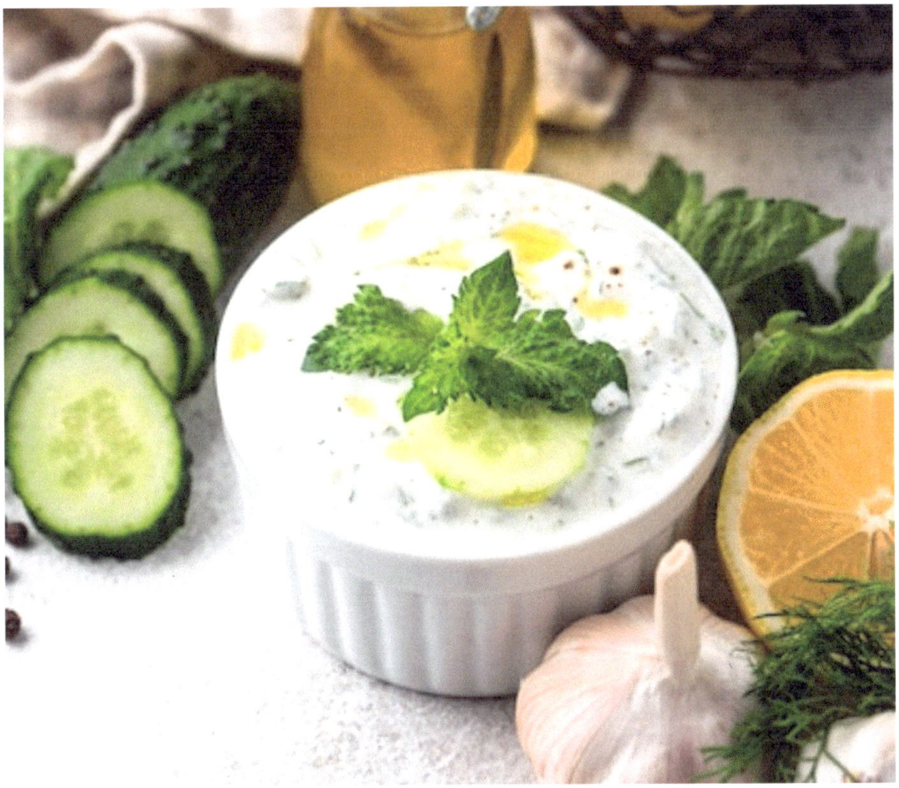

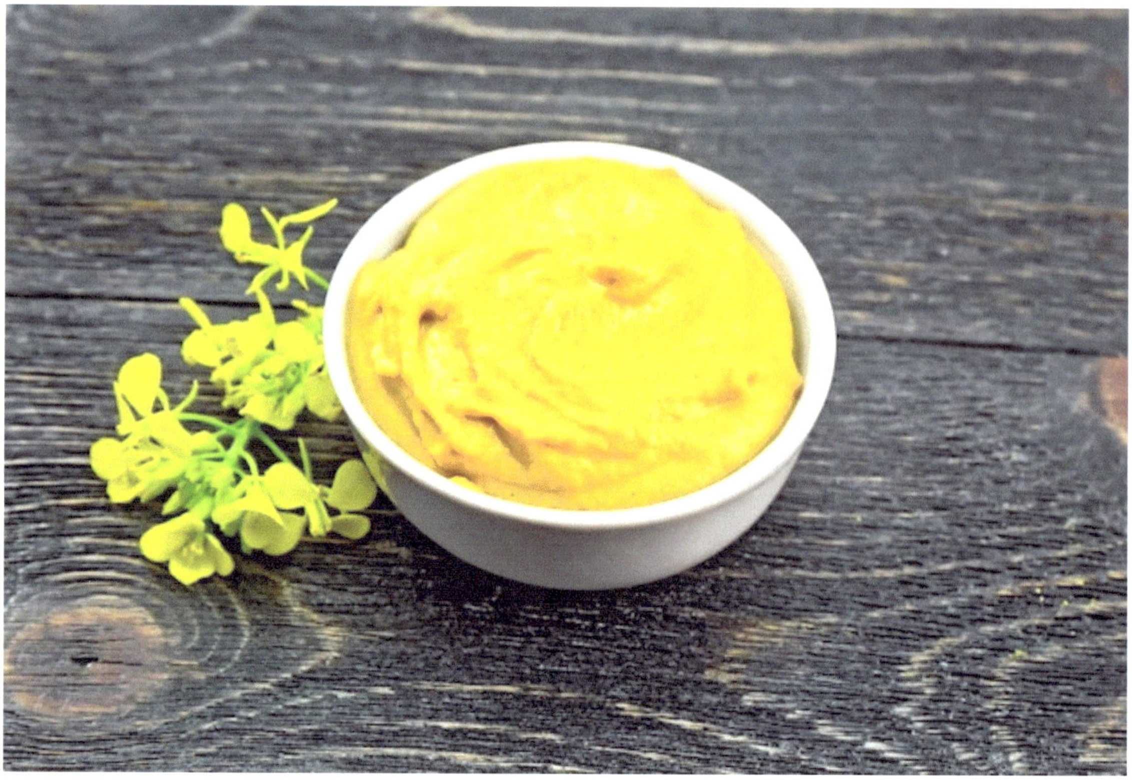

83. Mustard Dressing

Prep.Time: 5 min | **Cook Time:** 0 min | **Serving:** 4

Ingredients:

- 2 tablespoons Dijon mustard
- 2 tablespoons apple cider vinegar
- 2 tablespoons Greek yogurt (low-fat or non-fat)
- 1 tablespoon extra virgin olive oil
- 1 teaspoon sugar-free honey or maple syrup
- Salt and pepper to taste

Preparation:

1. In a small bowl, whisk together the Dijon mustard, apple cider vinegar, Greek yogurt, extra virgin olive oil, and sugar-free honey or maple syrup until well combined.
2. Season with salt and pepper according to taste.
3. Serve immediately over salads, grilled chicken, or as a dipping sauce for chicken tenders or vegetables.

Nutrient Facts (per serving):

- Calories: 50
- Carbohydrates: 2g
- Fat: 4g
- Protein: 2g

84. Mint Yogurt Sauce with Pomegranate

Prep.Time: 10 min

Cook Time: 0 min

Serving: 4

Ingredients:

- 1 cup Greek yogurt (low-fat or non-fat)
- 2 tablespoons chopped fresh mint leaves
- 2 tablespoons pomegranate arils
- 1 tablespoon lemon juice
- Salt to taste

Preparation:

1. In a mixing bowl, combine the Greek yogurt, chopped fresh mint leaves, pomegranate arils, and lemon juice.
2. Mix well until all ingredients are thoroughly combined.
3. Season with salt according to taste.
4. Serve chilled as a sauce for grilled lamb, chicken, or vegetables.

Nutrient Facts (per serving):

- Calories: 60
- Carbohydrates: 7g
- Fat: 3g
- Protein: 2g

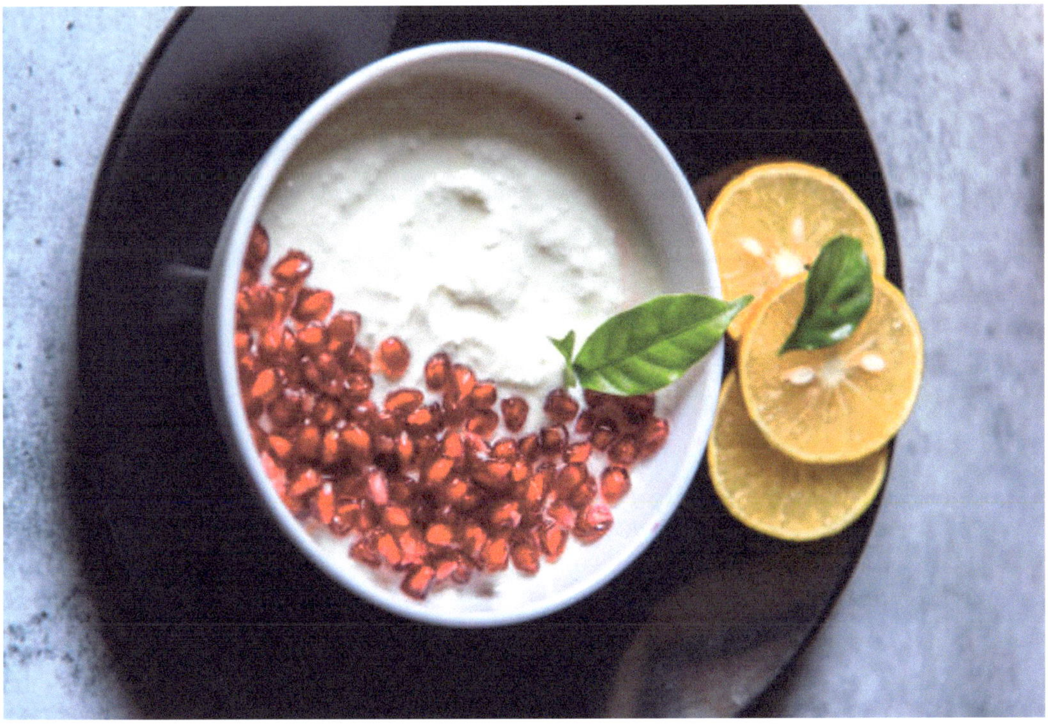

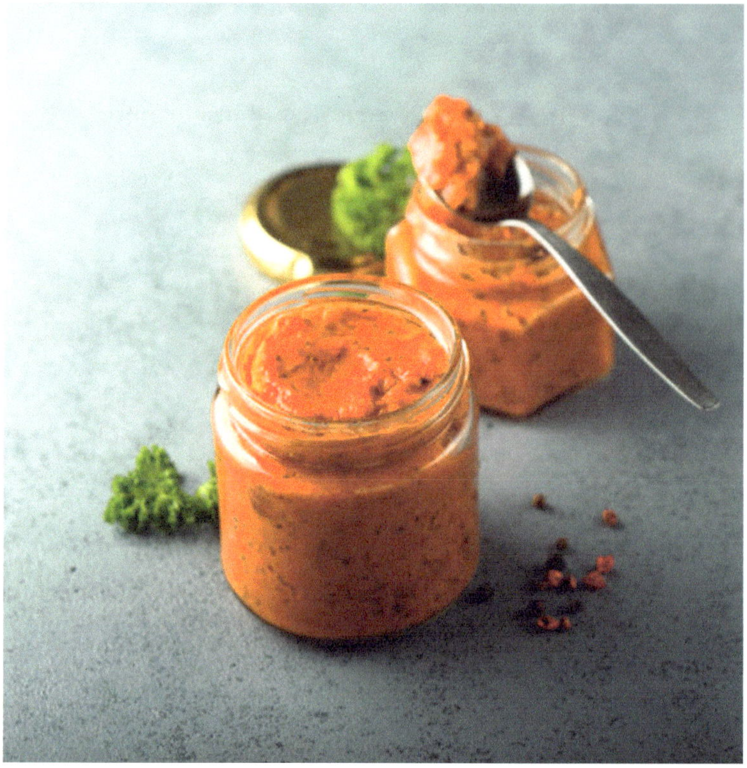

85. Roasted Eggplant and Red Pepper Dip

Prep.Time: 15 min

Cook Time: 30 min

Serving: 4

Ingredients:

- 1 medium eggplant, diced
- 1 red bell pepper, diced
- 2 cloves garlic, minced
- 2 tablespoons extra virgin olive oil
- 1 tablespoon lemon juice
- 1 tablespoon tahini (sesame seed paste)
- Salt and pepper to taste

Preparation:

1. Preheat the oven to 400°F (200°C).
2. In a large bowl, toss the diced eggplant, diced red bell pepper, minced garlic, and extra virgin olive oil until well coated.
3. Spread the mixture on a baking sheet in a single layer.
4. Roast in the preheated oven for about 25-30 minutes, or until the vegetables are tender and slightly caramelized, stirring halfway through.
5. Remove from the oven and let cool slightly.
6. In a food processor, combine the roasted vegetables, lemon juice, tahini, salt, and pepper.
7. Pulse until the mixture is smooth and creamy, scraping down the sides of the processor as needed.
8. Taste and adjust seasoning if necessary.
9. Transfer the roasted eggplant and red pepper dip to a serving bowl.
10. Serve chilled or at room temperature with pita bread, crackers, or vegetable sticks.

Nutrient Facts (per serving):

- Calories: 70
- Carbohydrates: 6g
- Fat: 5g
- Protein: 1g

86. Pumpkin Seed and Cilantro Lime Pesto

Prep.Time: 10 min | **Cook Time:** 0 min | **Serving:** 4

Ingredients:

- 1/2 cup pumpkin seeds (pepitas), toasted
- 1 cup fresh cilantro leaves
- 1/4 cup grated Parmesan cheese
- 2 cloves garlic, minced
- Zest and juice of 1 lime
- 1/4 cup extra virgin olive oil
- Salt and pepper to taste

Preparation:

1. In a food processor, combine the toasted pumpkin seeds, cilantro leaves, grated Parmesan cheese, minced garlic, lime zest, and lime juice.
2. Pulse until the mixture is coarsely chopped.
3. With the food processor running, slowly drizzle in the extra virgin olive oil until the pesto reaches your desired consistency.
4. Season with salt and pepper according to taste.
5. Transfer the pumpkin seed and cilantro lime pesto to a serving bowl.
6. Serve immediately tossed with cooked pasta, spread on sandwiches, or as a dip for vegetable sticks or crackers.

Nutrient Facts (per serving):

- Calories: 90
- Carbohydrates: 2g
- Fat: 8g
- Protein: 3g

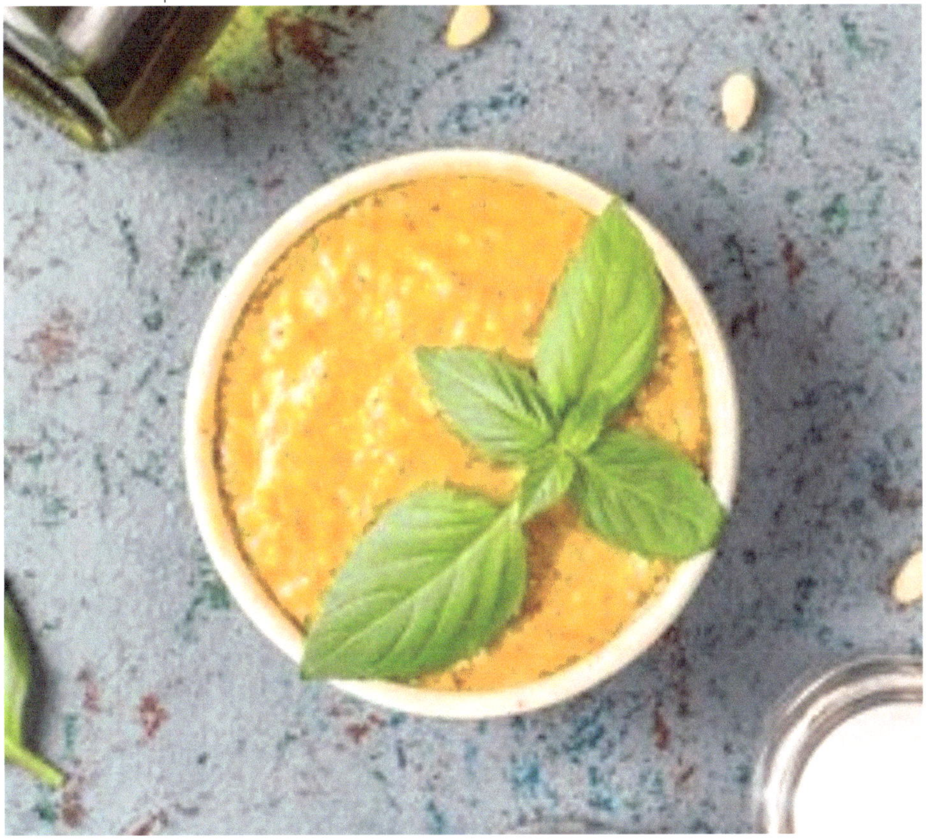

87. Cucumber Ranch Greek Yogurt Dip

Prep.Time: 10 min | **Cook Time:** 0 min | **Serving:** 4

Ingredients:

- 1 cup Greek yogurt (low-fat or non-fat)
- 1/2 cucumber, grated and excess moisture squeezed out
- 2 tablespoons chopped fresh dill
- 1 clove garlic, minced
- 1 tablespoon lemon juice
- Salt and pepper to taste

Preparation:

1. In a mixing bowl, combine the Greek yogurt, grated cucumber, chopped fresh dill, minced garlic, lemon juice, salt, and pepper.
2. Mix well until all ingredients are thoroughly combined.
3. Taste and adjust seasoning if necessary.
4. Serve chilled as a dip for vegetable sticks, pita chips, or as a sauce for grilled meats or falafel.

Nutrient Facts (per serving):

- Calories: 50
- Carbohydrates: 3g
- Fat: 3g
- Protein: 3g

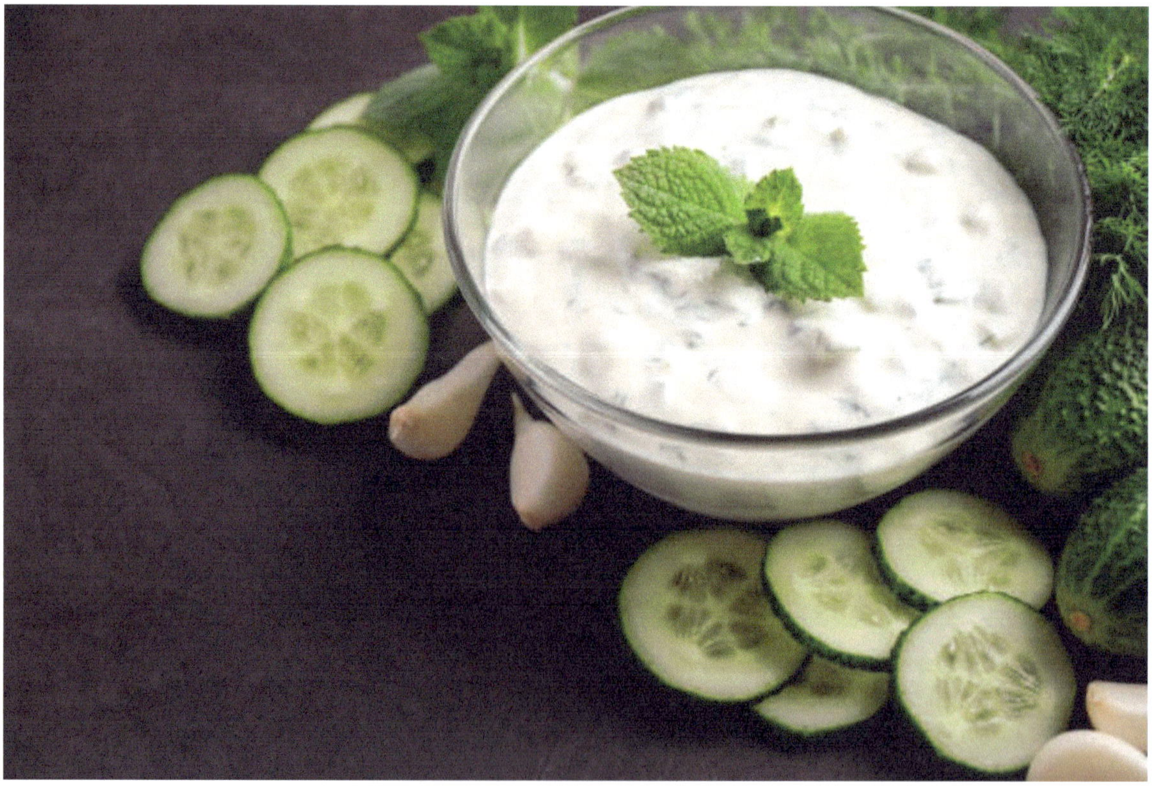

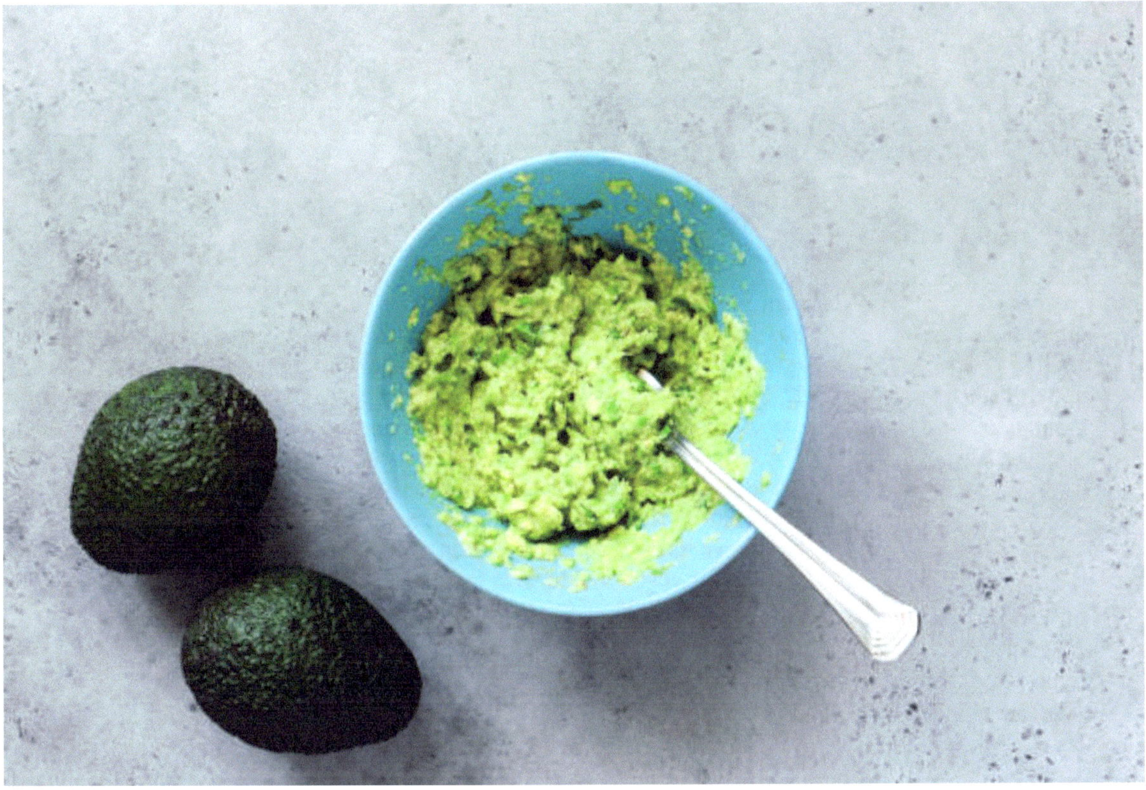

88. Avocado Chimichurri Sauce

Prep.Time: 10 min

Cook Time: 0 min

Serving: 4

Ingredients:

- 1 ripe avocado, peeled and pitted
- 1/4 cup chopped fresh parsley
- 2 tablespoons chopped fresh cilantro
- 2 tablespoons chopped fresh oregano
- 2 cloves garlic, minced
- 2 tablespoons red wine vinegar
- 1/4 cup extra virgin olive oil
- Salt and pepper to taste

Preparation:

1. In a food processor, combine the ripe avocado, chopped parsley, chopped cilantro, chopped oregano, minced garlic, red wine vinegar, and extra virgin olive oil.
2. Pulse until smooth and creamy, scraping down the sides of the processor as needed.
3. Season with salt and pepper according to taste.
4. Transfer the chimichurri sauce to a serving bowl.
5. Serve immediately as a sauce for grilled meats, seafood, or vegetables.

Nutrient Facts (per serving):

- Calories: 70
- Carbohydrates: 2g
- Fat: 7g
- Protein: 1g

89. Tomato Basil Pesto

Prep.Time:	Cook Time:	Serving:
10 min	0 min	4

Ingredients:

- 1 cup fresh basil leaves
- 1/4 cup pine nuts or walnuts
- 2 cloves garlic, minced
- 1/4 cup grated Parmesan cheese
- 1/4 cup extra virgin olive oil
- 1/2 cup diced tomatoes
- Salt and pepper to taste

Preparation:

1. In a food processor, combine the basil leaves, pine nuts or walnuts, minced garlic, grated Parmesan cheese, and extra virgin olive oil.
2. Pulse until smooth, scraping down the sides of the processor as needed.
3. Add the diced tomatoes to the mixture and pulse a few more times until the tomatoes are well incorporated but still slightly chunky.
4. Season with salt and pepper according to taste.
5. Transfer the tomato basil pesto to a serving bowl.
6. Serve immediately tossed with cooked pasta, spread on sandwiches, or as a dip for vegetable sticks or crackers.

Nutrient Facts (per serving):

- Calories: 110
- Carbohydrates: 2g
- Fat: 10g
- Protein: 2g

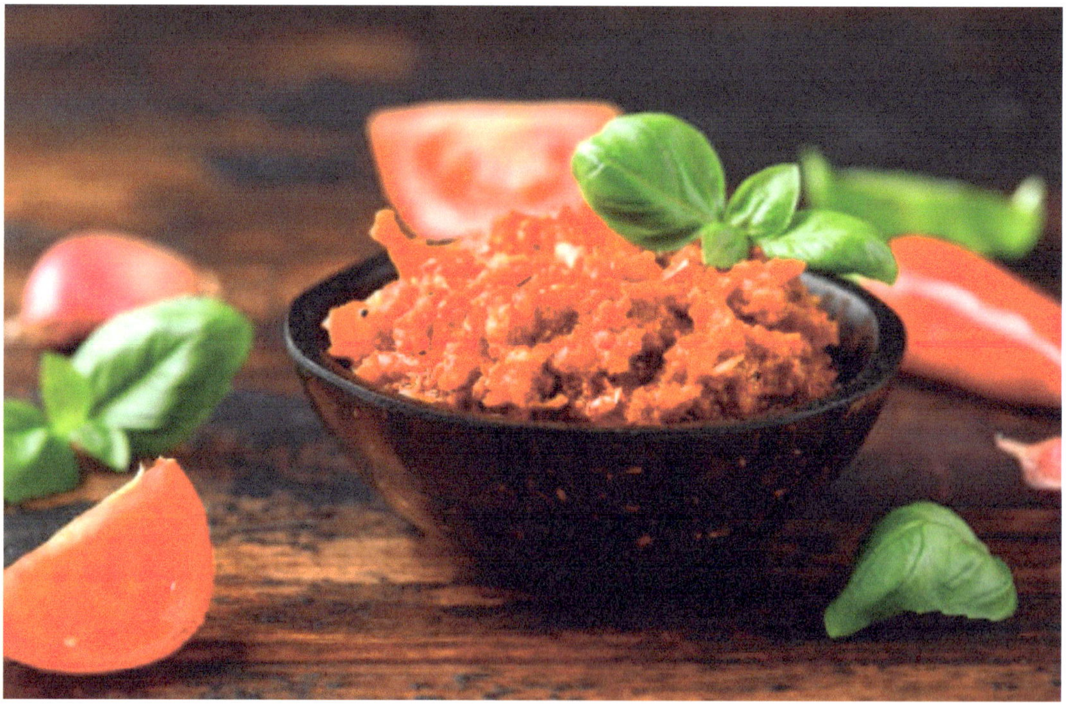

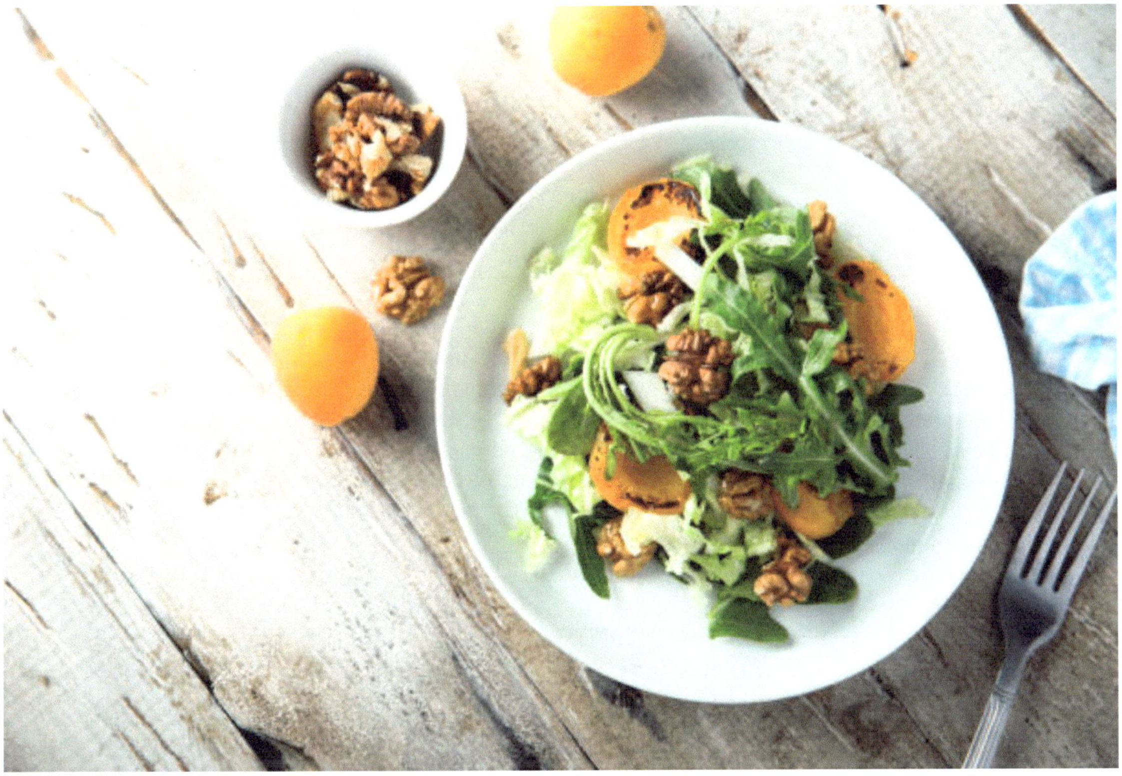

90. Lemon Walnut Vinaigrette

Prep.Time:	Cook Time:	Serving:
5 min	0 min	4

Ingredients:

- 1/4 cup walnut oil
- 2 tablespoons lemon juice
- 1 teaspoon Dijon mustard
- 1 teaspoon maple syrup
- 1 clove garlic, minced
- Salt and pepper to taste

Preparation:

1. In a small bowl, whisk together the walnut oil, lemon juice, Dijon mustard, maple syrup, minced garlic, salt, and pepper until well combined.
2. Taste and adjust seasoning if necessary.
3. Serve immediately over salads, roasted vegetables, or grilled meats.

Nutrient Facts (per serving):

- Calories: 80
- Carbohydrates: 2g
- Fat: 8g
- Protein: 1g

91. Cauliflower Tzatziki Sauce

Prep.Time: 15 min | **Cook Time:** 15 min | **Serving:** 4

Ingredients:

- 1 cup grated cauliflower
- 1/2 cup Greek yogurt (low-fat or non-fat)
- 1/4 cup grated cucumber, squeezed to remove excess moisture
- 1 clove garlic, minced
- 1 tablespoon chopped fresh dill
- 1 tablespoon lemon juice
- Salt and pepper to taste

Preparation:

1. In a skillet, sauté the grated cauliflower over medium heat for about 10-15 minutes, or until softened and slightly browned.
2. In a mixing bowl, combine the sautéed cauliflower, Greek yogurt, grated cucumber, minced garlic, chopped fresh dill, lemon juice, salt, and pepper.
3. Mix well until all ingredients are thoroughly combined.
4. Taste and adjust seasoning if necessary.
5. Serve chilled as a dip for vegetable sticks, pita chips, or as a sauce for grilled meats or falafel.

Nutrient Facts (per serving):

- Calories: 40
- Carbohydrates: 4g
- Fat: 2g
- Protein: 2g

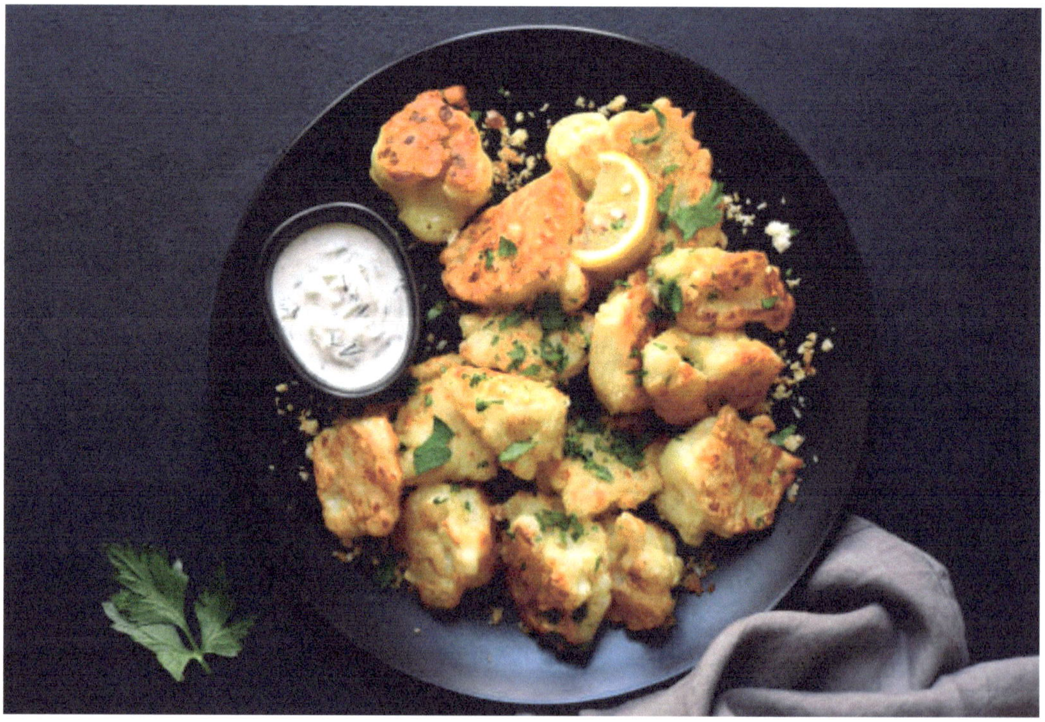

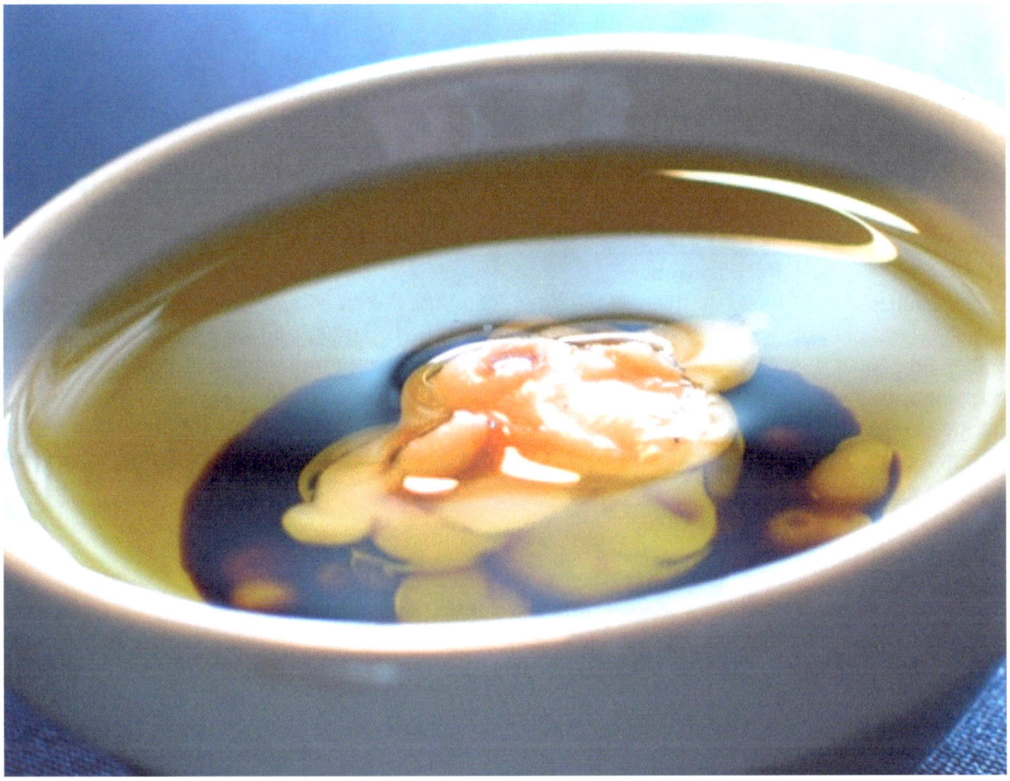

92. Sesame Soy Cilantro Dipping Sauce

Prep.Time: 5 min | **Cook Time:** 0 min | **Serving:** 4

Ingredients:

- 2 tablespoons soy sauce (low-sodium)
- 1 tablespoon rice vinegar
- 1 teaspoon sesame oil
- 1 teaspoon maple syrup
- 1 tablespoon chopped fresh cilantro
- 1 teaspoon sesame seeds (optional)
- 1 green onion, thinly sliced (optional)

Preparation:

1. In a small bowl, whisk together the soy sauce, rice vinegar, sesame oil, maple syrup, and chopped fresh cilantro until well combined.
2. If desired, garnish with sesame seeds and thinly sliced green onion.
3. Serve immediately as a dipping sauce for sushi, spring rolls, dumplings, or grilled meats and vegetables.

Nutrient Facts (per serving):

- Calories: 40
- Carbohydrates: 2g
- Fat: 3g
- Protein: 1g

93. Peach Jalapeño Salsa

Prep.Time: 15 min | **Cook Time:** 0 min | **Serving:** 4

Ingredients:

- 2 ripe peaches, diced
- 1 jalapeño pepper, seeded and finely chopped
- 1/4 cup red onion, finely chopped
- 2 tablespoons chopped fresh cilantro
- 1 tablespoon lime juice
- Salt and pepper to taste

Preparation:

1. In a mixing bowl, combine the diced peaches, chopped jalapeño pepper, chopped red onion, chopped cilantro, and lime juice.
2. Mix well until all ingredients are thoroughly combined.
3. Season with salt and pepper according to taste.
4. Let the salsa sit for about 10 minutes to allow the flavors to meld.
5. Serve chilled with tortilla chips, grilled chicken or fish, or as a topping for tacos.

Nutrient Facts (per serving):

- Calories: 40
- Carbohydrates: 10g
- Fat: 0g
- Protein: 1g

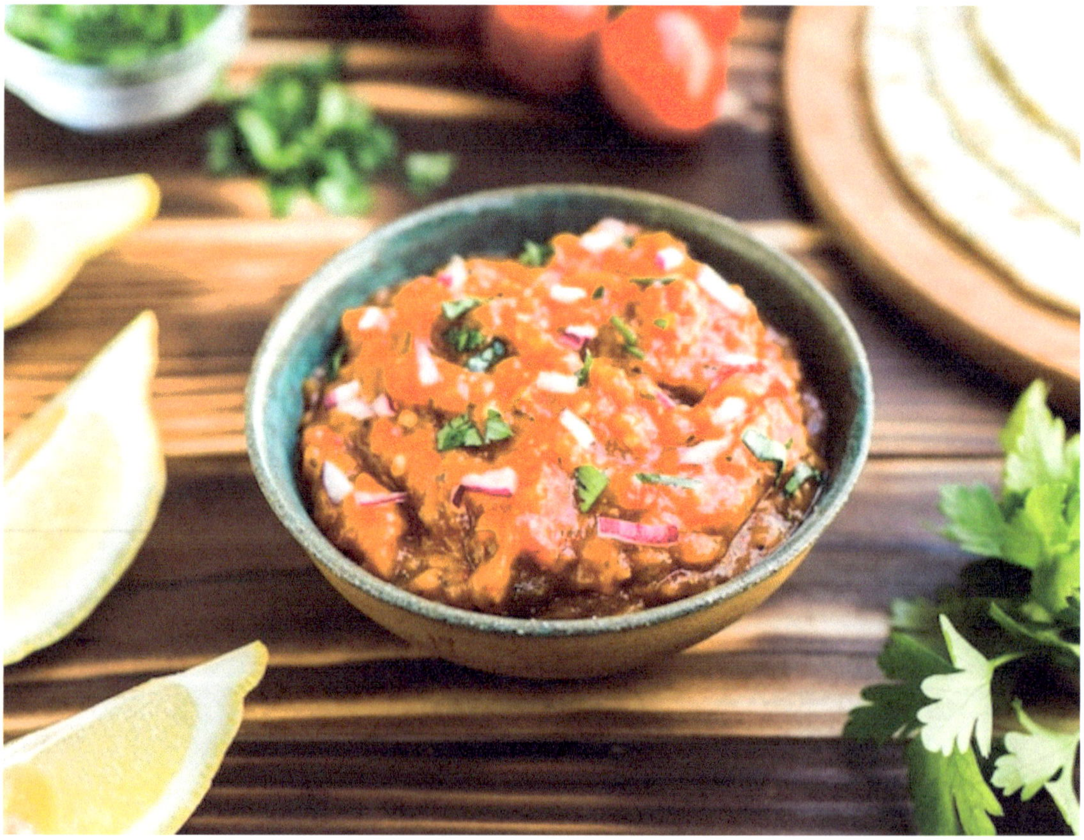

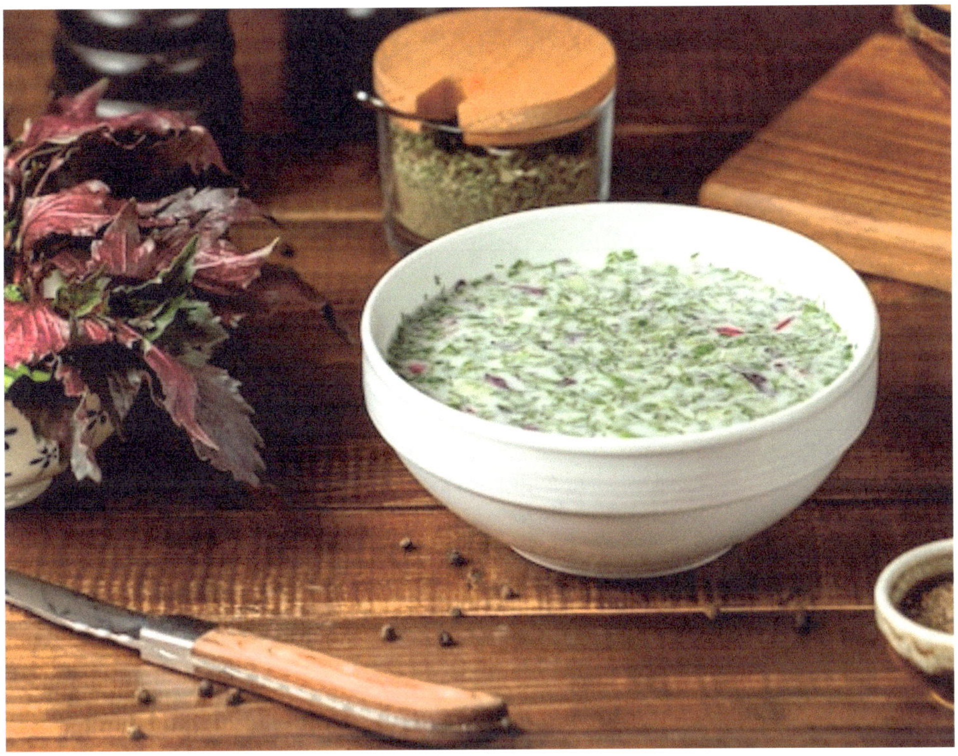

94. Cilantro Lime Greek Yogurt Dressing

Prep.Time: 5 min

Cook Time: 0 min

Serving: 4

Ingredients:

- 1/2 cup Greek yogurt (low-fat or non-fat)
- 2 tablespoons chopped fresh cilantro
- 1 tablespoon lime juice
- 1 clove garlic, minced
- Salt and pepper to taste

Preparation:

1. In a mixing bowl, combine the Greek yogurt, chopped cilantro, lime juice, minced garlic, salt, and pepper.
2. Mix well until all ingredients are thoroughly combined.
3. Taste and adjust seasoning if necessary.
4. Serve immediately as a dressing for salads, grilled vegetables, or tacos.

Nutrient Facts (per serving):

- Calories: 60
- Carbohydrates: 4g
- Fat: 3g
- Protein: 4g

95. Sun-Dried Tomato and Basil Hummus

Prep.Time: 10 min | **Cook Time:** 0 min | **Serving:** 4

Ingredients:

- 1 can (15 ounces) chickpeas (garbanzo beans), drained and rinsed
- 1/4 cup sun-dried tomatoes (packed in oil), drained
- 2 tablespoons chopped fresh basil
- 1 clove garlic, minced
- 2 tablespoons lemon juice
- 2 tablespoons extra virgin olive oil
- Salt and pepper to taste

Preparation:

1. In a food processor, combine the chickpeas, sun-dried tomatoes, chopped basil, minced garlic, lemon juice, extra virgin olive oil, salt, and pepper.
2. Pulse until smooth and creamy, scraping down the sides of the processor as needed.
3. If the hummus is too thick, add water, one tablespoon at a time, until it reaches your desired consistency.
4. Taste and adjust seasoning if necessary.
5. Transfer the sun-dried tomato and basil hummus to a serving bowl.
6. Serve immediately as a dip for pita bread, vegetable sticks, or as a spread for sandwiches.

Nutrient Facts (per serving):

- Calories: 90
- Carbohydrates: 6g
- Fat: 6g
- Protein: 3g

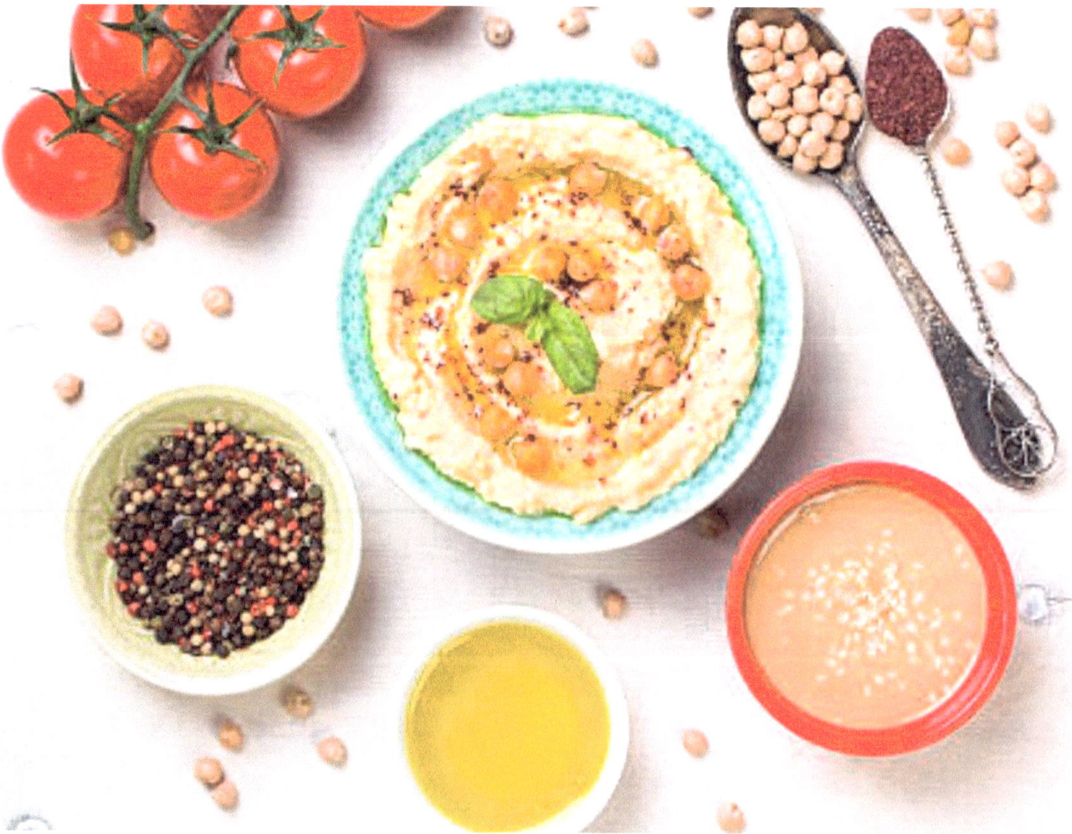

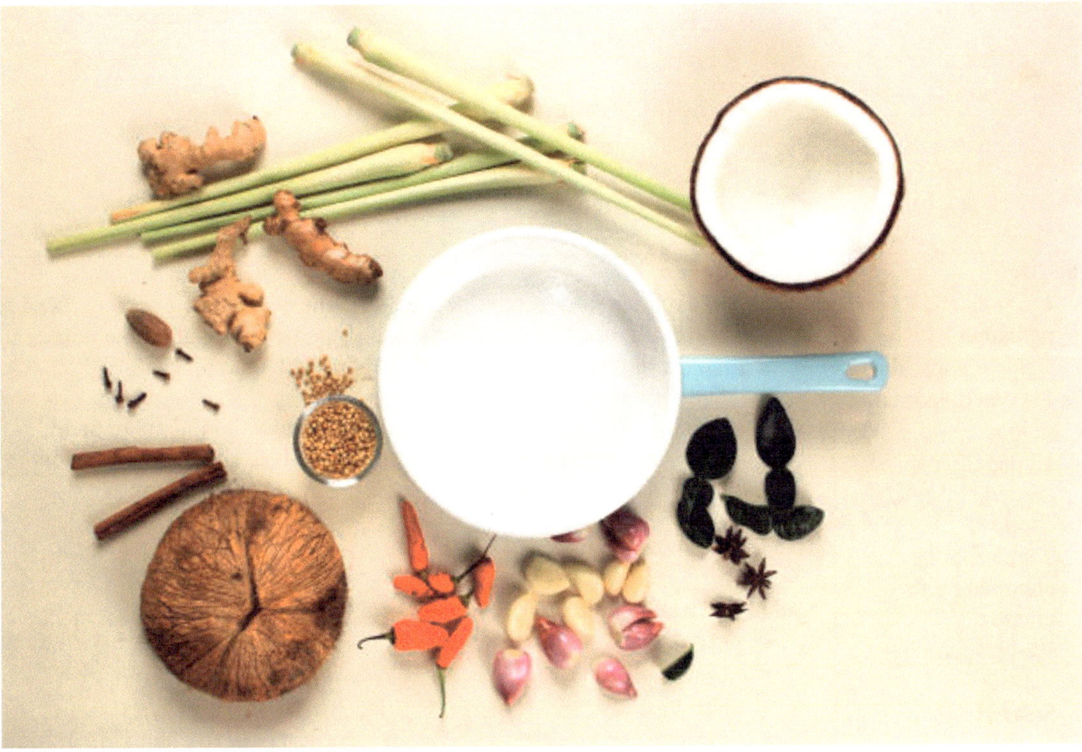

96. Coconut Aminos Garlic Ginger Sauce

Prep.Time: 5 min	Cook Time: 5 min	Serving: 4

Ingredients:

- 1/4 cup coconut aminos
- 1 tablespoon rice vinegar
- 1 teaspoon sesame oil
- 1 teaspoon minced fresh ginger
- 2 cloves garlic, minced
- Pinch of red pepper flakes (optional)

Preparation:

1. In a small saucepan, combine the coconut aminos, rice vinegar, sesame oil, minced ginger, minced garlic, and red pepper flakes (if using).
2. Cook over low heat for about 5 minutes, stirring occasionally, until the sauce has slightly thickened and the flavors have melded.
3. Remove from heat and let cool slightly before serving.
4. Serve warm or at room temperature as a dipping sauce for spring rolls, dumplings, or grilled meats and vegetables.

Nutrient Facts (per serving):

- Calories: 30
- Carbohydrates: 4g
- Fat: 1g
- Protein: 1g

97. Spicy Pineapple Mango Salsa

Prep.Time: 15 min | **Cook Time:** 0 min | **Serving:** 4

Ingredients:

- 1 cup diced pineapple
- 1 ripe mango, diced
- 1/4 cup diced red onion
- 1 jalapeño pepper, seeded and finely chopped
- 2 tablespoons chopped fresh cilantro
- 1 tablespoon lime juice
- Salt to taste

Preparation:

1. In a mixing bowl, combine the diced pineapple, diced mango, diced red onion, chopped jalapeño pepper, chopped cilantro, and lime juice.
2. Mix well until all ingredients are thoroughly combined.
3. Season with salt according to taste.
4. Let the salsa sit for about 10 minutes to allow the flavors to meld.
5. Serve chilled with tortilla chips, grilled fish or chicken, or as a topping for tacos or salads.

Nutrient Facts (per serving):

- Calories: 45
- Carbohydrates: 12g
- Fat: 0g
- Protein: 1g

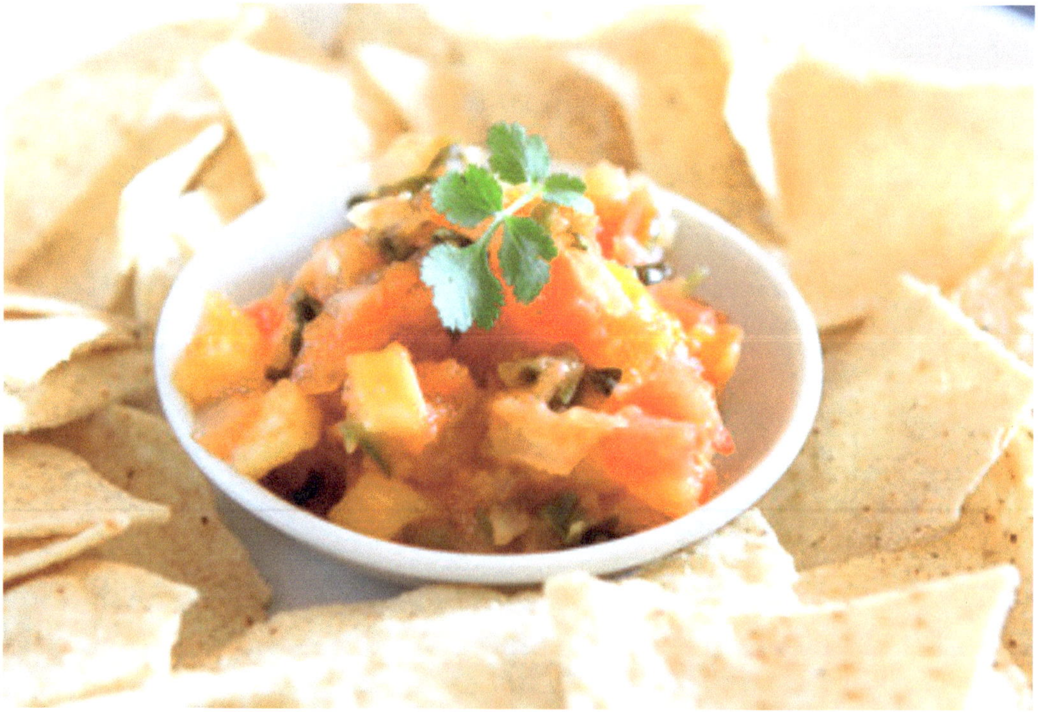

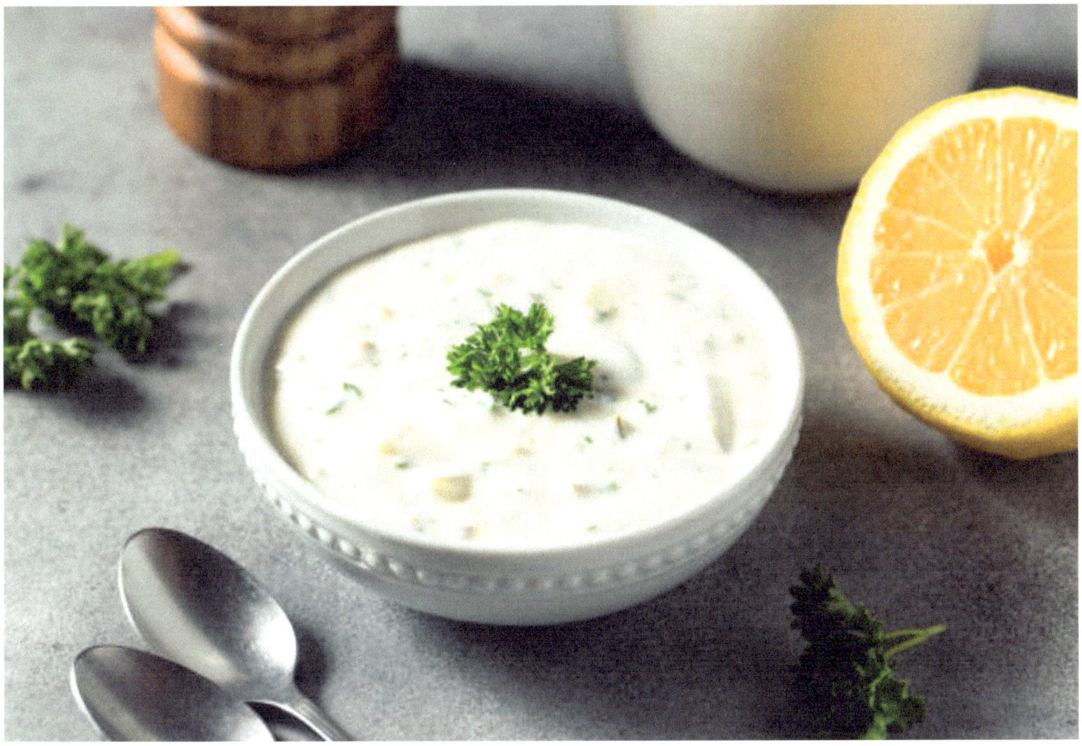

98. Lemon Herb Aioli

Prep.Time: 10 min | **Cook Time:** 0 min | **Serving:** 4

Ingredients:

- 1 cup mayonnaise (low-fat or regular)
- 2 cloves garlic, minced
- Zest and juice of 1 lemon
- 2 tablespoons chopped fresh herbs (such as parsley, basil, or chives)
- Salt and pepper to taste

Preparation:

1. In a mixing bowl, combine the mayonnaise, minced garlic, lemon zest, lemon juice, and chopped fresh herbs.
2. Mix well until all ingredients are thoroughly combined.
3. Season with salt and pepper according to taste.
4. Serve immediately as a dipping sauce for roasted vegetables, seafood, or as a spread for sandwiches or burgers.

Nutrient Facts (per serving):

- Calories: 90
- Carbohydrates: 1g
- Fat: 10g
- Protein: 1g

99. Kale Cashew Cream

Prep.Time:	Cook Time:	Serving:
15 min	10 min	4

Ingredients:

- 2 cups kale leaves, stems removed
- 1 cup raw cashews, soaked in hot water for 30 minutes and drained
- 2 cloves garlic
- Juice of 1 lemon
- 1/4 cup water
- Salt and pepper to taste

Preparation:

1. In a food processor or blender, combine kale leaves, soaked cashews, garlic cloves, lemon juice, and water.
2. Blend until smooth and creamy, scraping down the sides as needed. If the mixture is too thick, add more water as needed to reach the desired consistency.
3. Season with salt and pepper to taste.
4. Serve the kale cashew cream as a sauce for pasta, as a spread on sandwiches or wraps, or as a dip for raw vegetables.

Nutrient Facts (per serving):

- Calories: 160
- Carbohydrates: 10g
- Fat: 12g
- Protein: 5g

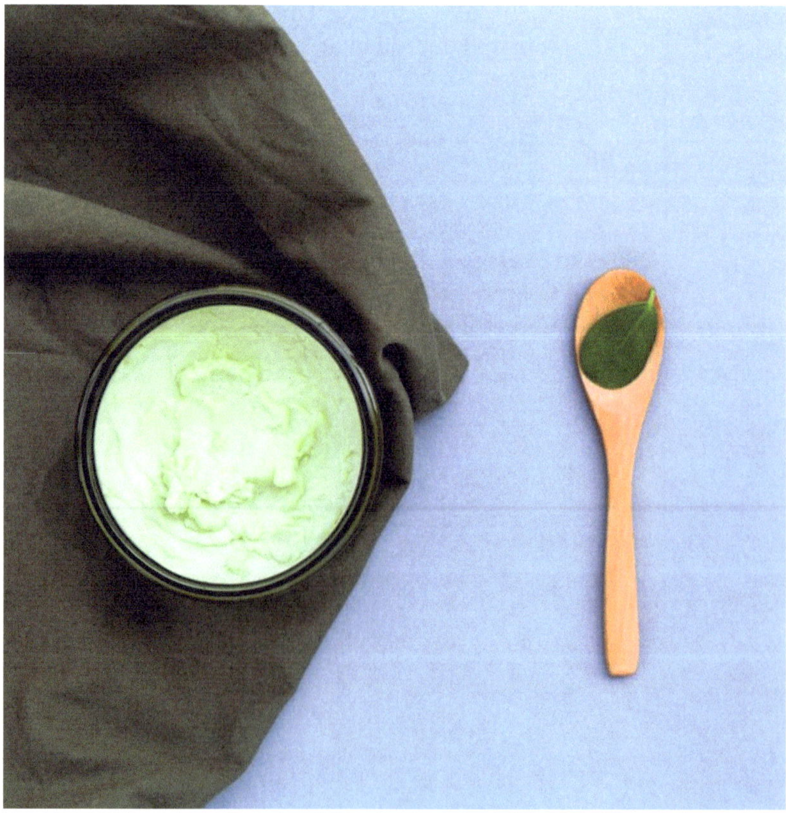

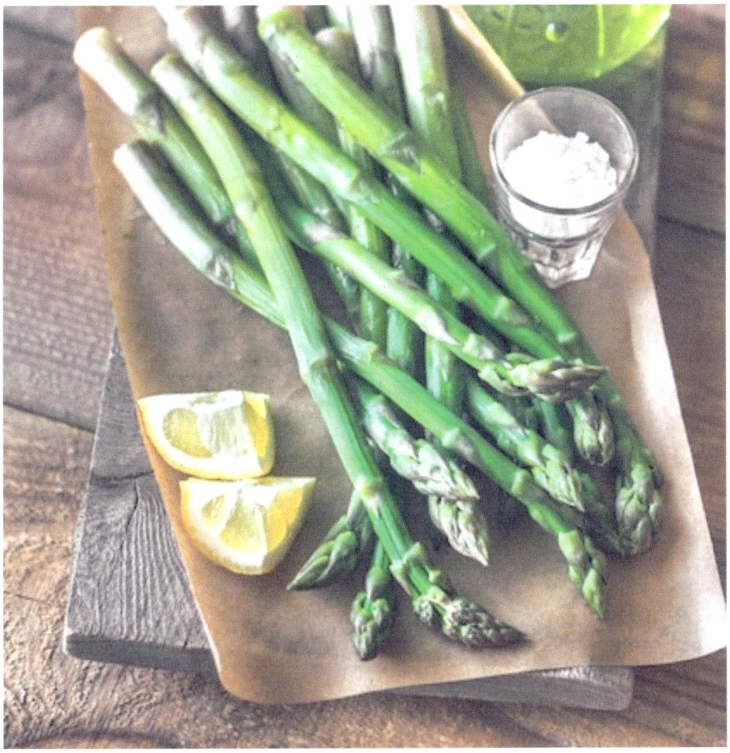

100. Asparagus Lemon Dill Dressing

Prep.Time: 10 min

Cook Time: 5 min

Serving: 4

Ingredients:

- 1 bunch asparagus, trimmed and steamed
- Zest and juice of 1 lemon
- 2 tablespoons fresh dill, chopped
- 1/4 cup olive oil
- Salt and pepper to taste

Preparation:

1. In a blender or food processor, combine steamed asparagus, lemon zest, lemon juice, chopped dill, olive oil, salt, and pepper.
2. Blend until smooth and creamy.
3. Taste and adjust seasoning if necessary.
4. Serve the asparagus lemon dill dressing over salads, grilled vegetables, or as a dip for crudité.

Nutrient Facts (per serving):

- Calories: 70
- Carbohydrates: 5g
- Fat: 5g
- Protein: 2g

Sharing Your Culinary Journey

Now that you've mastered the art of creating delicious, diabetes-friendly meals, it's time to share your newfound culinary wisdom with others who are on the same path. By leaving your honest review of the "Type 2 Diabetes Cookbook: Beginner's Quick & Easy Recipes for Delicious Diabetes Diets" by Lily Anders on Amazon, you'll guide fellow food enthusiasts to a resource that can transform their dining table and health.

Your insights and experiences are invaluable, offering a beacon to those navigating their diet amidst diabetes. Whether it was a specific recipe that became your go-to, a tip that changed how you approach cooking, or the overall ease and enjoyment you found in these pages, your feedback is a gift that keeps on giving.

Thank you for contributing to a community of knowledge and support. The journey towards healthy eating and diabetes management thrives on shared discoveries and successes. By passing on your review, you're not just recommending a book—you're enriching lives with the joy of cooking and the empowerment of dietary control.

To leave your review, just follow this link:

https://www.amazon.com/review/create-review/?ie=UTF8&channel=glance-detail&asin=1963939344

Together, we're keeping the passion for healthy, joyful eating alive, one review at a time. Your support makes all the difference, not just to us, but to every reader and cook who seeks to balance their love for food with their health needs.

- With heartfelt thanks,

Lily Anders

Conclusion

In conclusion, this book transcends the traditional approach to managing diabetes through diet alone, offering a comprehensive guide that empowers individuals with diabetes to navigate their condition with knowledge and precision. Through 300 carefully crafted recipes, we explore the importance of balancing nutrient intake and the vital role of consistent meal planning. Each recipe is not just a set of instructions but a building block towards a healthier life, tailored to the unique needs of those managing diabetes.

As we close this journey of understanding and adaptation, remember that managing diabetes is not just about adhering to dietary restrictions or grappling with numbers—it is about reclaiming control of your health and life. These recipes are designed not only to meet specific nutritional needs but also to delight the palate, proving that a diabetes-conscious diet can be as delicious as it is nutritious.

Embrace these culinary tools as your allies in the pursuit of wellness. Let each meal enrich your body and spirit, and may the knowledge contained in this book guide you toward a balanced, joyful, and healthy life with diabetes. Here's to finding pleasure in every bite and strength in every challenge. Cheers to your health and happiness on this flavorful journey!

Made in the USA
Monee, IL
13 September 2026

62976621R00074